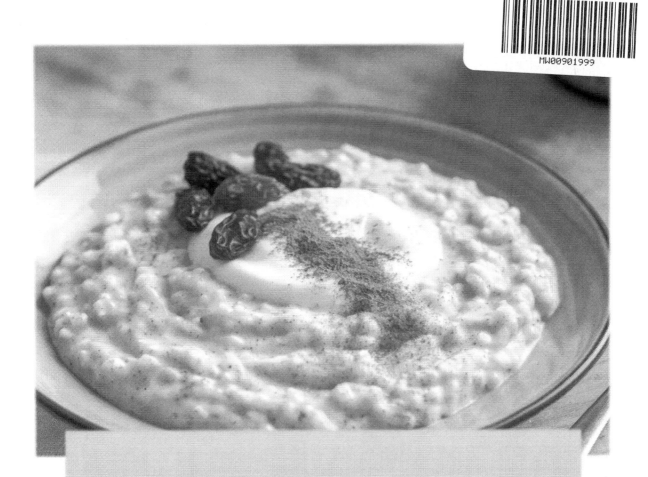

Dysphagia Cookbook For Beginners

Nutritious And Easy Recipes With Meal Plan
For Chewing And Swallowing Difficulties

Brenda R. Willis

Dysphagia cookbook for beginners

Table of Contents

Dysphagia cookbook for beginners

Dysphagia cookbook for beginners

Dysphagia cookbook for beginners

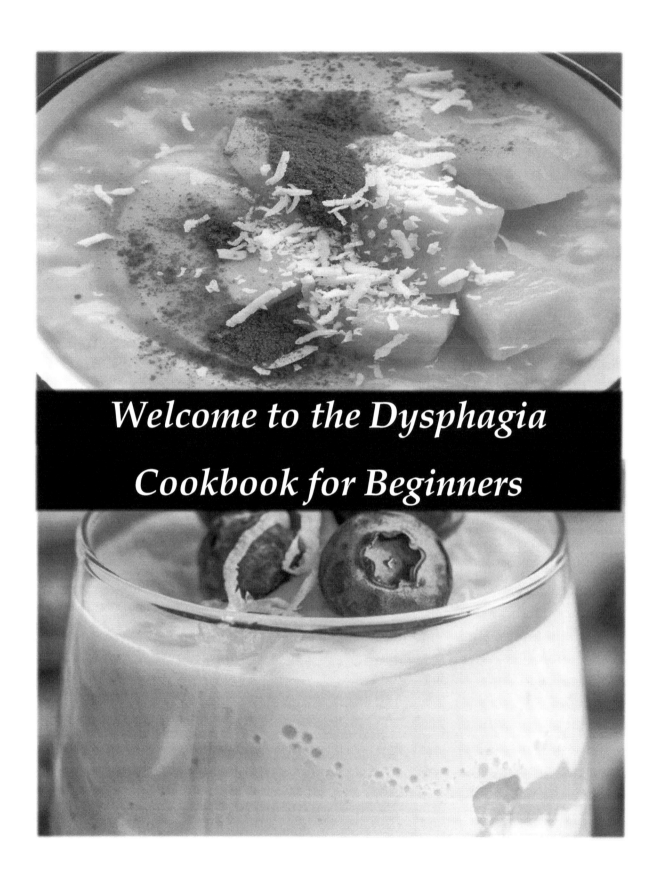

Welcome to the Dysphagia Cookbook for Beginners

Preface

My passion has always been to help people improve their health through the food they eat. Over the years, I've come to understand just how much we rely on the ability to enjoy food—not just for nutrition but for connection, comfort, and joy. But for individuals with dysphagia, eating can become a challenge that impacts every aspect of daily life.

This cookbook is inspired from my desire to provide a resource that makes navigating a dysphagia diet easier, more manageable, and most importantly—enjoyable. I have worked closely with individuals facing this condition, seeing firsthand the struggles they endure. I've met people who felt that their food choices were suddenly stripped down to bland, tasteless options, and caregivers overwhelmed by the complexity of dietary restrictions. This experience drove me to create this book.

In my work, I've come to understand the critical balance between safety and nutrition, but also the need to preserve the pleasure in eating. A meal should never feel like a burden, and no one should have to give up the satisfaction of good food simply because they have swallowing difficulties. With the right tools, I believe anyone can prepare meals that are not only safe but delicious and nourishing.

This book is designed to guide you step by step, whether you're just starting to adjust to a dysphagia diet or you've been managing it for years. Each recipe is crafted with a focus on nutrition, texture, and flavor, to ensure that you or your loved one can still enjoy the variety that food offers while maintaining safety.

It's my hope that this cookbook helps to lift some of the burdens associated with dysphagia.

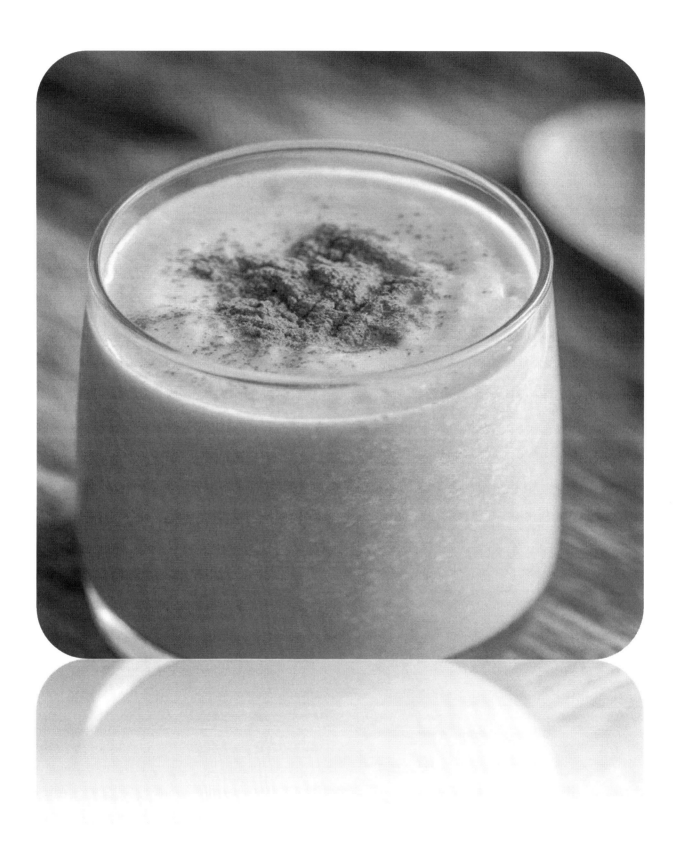

Introduction

Welcome to the Dysphagia Cookbook for Beginners

Eating is such a fundamental part of life. It brings people together, provides comfort, and nourishes our bodies. But for those living with dysphagia, eating can feel more like a challenge than a source of enjoyment. This cookbook was created with you in mind—to make navigating your new dietary needs simpler, safer, and yes, even more enjoyable.

What to Expect from This Book

This book is more than just a collection of recipes. It's your guide to reclaiming the pleasure of eating while managing dysphagia. Whether you're new to these dietary changes or have been adjusting for some time, you'll find everything you need here easy-to-understand explanations of Dysphagia-friendly foods to practical advice for caregivers and loved ones.

Inside, you'll discover:

- **Three levels of dysphagia diets**: We'll break down each level, from pureed foods to soft solids, so you can confidently prepare meals that meet your or your loved one's needs.

- **Nutritious, flavorful recipes**: Every recipe is designed with care, ensuring that you don't sacrifice nutrition or flavor. Whether it's a comforting bowl of creamy soup or a soft, satisfying main course, there's something for every mealtime.

- **Tools and techniques**: Learn how to modify everyday meals to fit dysphagia requirements, and discover the grocery shopping guide that can make food preparation easier and faster.

by the whole family, making mealtime less stressful.

How to Use this Cookbook

Finding dysphagia-friendly foods can feel overwhelming at first, but this cookbook is structured to guide you through it step by step. Here's how to make the most of it:

1. Start with the Basics: If you're new to a dysphagia diet, begin by exploring the chapters 1 that explain all you need to know about dysphagia.

2. Select Recipes Based on Texture: The recipes are organized according to the dysphagia diet levels. If you're following a Level 1 diet (pureed foods), you can easily find recipes that suit your needs, and the same goes for Levels 2 and 3. This structure ensures that you're always preparing meals that are safe and enjoyable.

3. Meal Planning Made Simple: With breakfast, lunch, dinner, snacks, and even desserts covered, you can plan out a week's worth of meals without worry. Many recipes are versatile enough to be enjoyed

4. Customize and Modify: Feel free to modify recipes to fit your specific tastes or dietary needs. I've provided plenty of variations and substitutions where possible, so that you can adapt the meals to your preferences.

Whether you are preparing meals for yourself or a loved one, I hope this cookbook serves as a trusted companion. You deserve meals that are safe, nutritious, and above all, enjoyable. Welcome to a new chapter in your eating journey—let's bring the joy back to the table!

Dysphagia cookbook for beginners

Chapter 1

Understanding Dysphagia

What is Dysphagia?

Dysphagia is a medical condition that refers to difficulty swallowing. It can affect people of all ages but is more common in older adults or individuals with certain neurological or structural conditions. Swallowing is a complex process involving the mouth, throat, and esophagus, and dysphagia occurs when there is a disruption in any part of this process, making it hard to move food, liquids, or even saliva from the mouth to the stomach.

Why Is Dysphagia Serious?

Dysphagia can lead to malnutrition, dehydration, and a condition known as aspiration—where food or liquids enter the airway instead of the esophagus, leading to pneumonia or other respiratory issues. It can also severely impact the quality of life, making mealtimes stressful and frustrating. Managing dysphagia often involves modifying food textures and liquid consistencies to make swallowing safer. This is where a dysphagia diet comes into play, offering options to ensure individuals still receive the necessary nutrients without the risk of choking or aspiration.

Let explain more about Swallowing Difficulties for deep understanding

Swallowing is a complex process that involves the coordination of various muscles and nerves in the mouth, throat, and esophagus. It's something most of us do without much thought, yet for those with swallowing difficulties, or dysphagia, it can be a daunting and even dangerous task. Swallowing begins in the mouth, where food is chewed and mixed with saliva to form a manageable texture. This is known as the **oral phase.** Once the food is ready, the tongue pushes it toward the back of the mouth, initiating the **pharyngeal phase**, where it passes through the throat. This is followed by the **esophageal phase**, during which food moves down the esophagus and into the stomach.

Each phase of swallowing relies on precise timing and strength. In individuals with dysphagia, disruptions can occur at any point, causing a range of problems. Some people may have difficulty chewing and preparing food for swallowing, while others might find it challenging to move food past the throat. For some, the issue arises in the **esophagus**, where food gets stuck or moves too slowly toward the stomach. These disruptions not only make eating and drinking more difficult but also pose serious health risks.

One of the most common issues in swallowing difficulties is a delay or inability to trigger the swallowing reflex. In healthy swallowing, once food reaches the back of the throat, the brain sends signals to close off the airway, preventing food or liquid from entering the lungs. However, in those with dysphagia, this reflex may be weakened or slow, increasing the risk of aspiration. **Aspiration** occurs when food, liquid, or saliva accidentally enters the airway, which can lead to serious complications like pneumonia or chronic lung infections. This makes swallowing difficulties a potentially life-threatening condition if not managed properly.

Another factor that can complicate swallowing is a **lack of coordination** between the muscles in the mouth, throat, and esophagus. This can result from neurological conditions such as stroke, Parkinson's disease, or multiple sclerosis, where nerve damage impairs muscle control. In these cases, individuals might have difficulty forming a cohesive bolus, the term for the chewed food that is swallowed. When the muscles don't work in harmony, the bolus may not move smoothly through the throat and into the esophagus, causing choking, gagging, or the sensation of food being stuck.

Weakness in the muscles responsible for swallowing is another common problem. As people age, or in individuals with certain medical conditions, the muscles can lose strength, making it hard to push food through the pharynx and into the esophagus. This often results in the need to swallow multiple times to clear food from the mouth and throat. If food or liquid stays in the throat for too long, there is an increased risk of aspiration. Over time, these repeated efforts to swallow can lead to fatigue during meals, causing individuals to eat less and eventually leading to malnutrition.

Causes and Symptoms of Dysphagia

Dysphagia, or difficulty swallowing, can arise from a variety of causes that affect the mouth, throat, or esophagus. These causes can be broadly categorized into **neurological, structural, or muscular**

origins, though sometimes a combination of factors may be involved.

One of the most common causes is **neurological damage**. Conditions such as stroke, Parkinson's disease, multiple sclerosis, ALS (Amyotrophic Lateral Sclerosis), and dementia can impair the brain's ability to control the muscles involved in swallowing. In these cases, the nerves responsible for coordinating the swallowing process may become damaged or weakened, leading to difficulty in managing food or liquids in the mouth and throat. For people with such conditions, dysphagia can be a long-term issue that requires ongoing management. Brain or spinal cord injuries can also disrupt the neurological pathways needed for swallowing, making it difficult for individuals to complete the action smoothly and safely.

Another cause is **muscle weakness** or dysfunction. The muscles involved in swallowing need to be strong and coordinated for the process to work properly. As people age, the muscles in the throat and esophagus may weaken,

15

resulting in a higher risk of dysphagia. Certain muscular diseases, such as myasthenia gravis or muscular dystrophy, can also impair the body's ability to contract the necessary muscles effectively. In such cases, even forming a proper bolus (the chewed mass of food ready for swallowing) can become difficult, and moving it smoothly down the throat and esophagus becomes a challenge.

Structural abnormalities in the esophagus or throat can also lead to dysphagia. Some individuals may experience narrowing of the esophagus, known as strictures, which can make it harder for food to pass through. This narrowing can result from conditions like GERD (gastroesophageal reflux disease), where stomach acid repeatedly irritates the lining of the esophagus, causing inflammation and scar tissue. In more severe cases, tumors in the esophagus or throat—whether benign or malignant—can obstruct the normal passage of food and liquids, resulting in dysphagia. Surgical interventions in the head, neck, or throat, particularly for cancer, can also alter the anatomy, making swallowing more difficult.

Infections and inflammation can also contribute to dysphagia. For example, esophagitis, an inflammation of the esophagus, can make swallowing painful and difficult. This can be caused by infections, such as fungal infections in immunocompromised individuals, or by prolonged use of medications that irritate the esophagus. In rare cases, autoimmune diseases like scleroderma, which cause hardening and tightening of tissues, can lead to esophageal dysfunction and swallowing issues.

The symptoms of dysphagia can vary depending on the underlying cause and the severity of the condition. One of the most common symptoms is difficulty starting the swallowing process, particularly with solid foods. Individuals might notice a feeling of food being stuck in the throat or chest, or they may struggle to get food down smoothly. This can lead to coughing or choking during or after eating, especially with liquids or more solid textures. Some may experience pain when swallowing,

16

known as odynophagia, which can further complicate mealtime.

Another key symptom is *regurgitation*, where food or liquids come back up after swallowing, often accompanied by a sensation of food being stuck. In some cases, food or drink may enter the airway instead of the esophagus, leading to aspiration. Aspiration is particularly dangerous, as it can cause food or liquid to enter the lungs, leading to respiratory infections such as pneumonia. Recurrent respiratory issues or frequent pneumonia can be a sign of untreated dysphagia.

Also, **drooling or difficulty managing saliva** can also be a symptom of dysphagia, particularly in individuals with neurological causes of the condition. When swallowing becomes impaired, excess saliva may not be swallowed properly, leading to drooling or the accumulation of saliva in the mouth.

Importance of a Modified Diet

The importance of a modified diet for someone with dysphagia goes far beyond simply changing the texture of food. When I first encountered the reality of dysphagia, I saw how something as fundamental as eating—something most of us take for granted—became a source of stress, fear, and frustration. Every meal was a challenge, with the constant risk of choking or food going down the wrong way. Watching a loved one face these struggles, I realized how essential it is to ensure that food is not only safe to swallow but still enjoyable and nutritious.

For anyone managing dysphagia, a modified diet is much more than a recommendation; it's a necessity for safety. When food or liquid doesn't go down properly, it can enter the airway instead of the esophagus, leading to aspiration. Aspiration can cause respiratory infections like pneumonia, which can be life-threatening. This is why the texture of the food matters so much. By preparing foods that are smoother, softer, or easier to chew, we significantly reduce the chances of something going wrong. It's about creating peace of mind, knowing that every bite is safer.

But safety isn't the only thing that matters. Nutrition is key. When swallowing becomes difficult, many people eat less to avoid the discomfort or fear of choking, which can lead to weight loss, malnutrition, and dehydration. A modified diet is designed to keep that from happening. By making small adjustments—like blending vegetables into a puree or thickening drinks—we can ensure that someone with dysphagia still gets all the essential nutrients they need. Meals that are tailored for easier swallowing don't have to be bland or boring; they can be just as satisfying and delicious as any other meal, and they can help maintain strength, energy, and overall health.

Perhaps one of the most profound impacts I've seen with a modified diet is how it restores a sense of normalcy and enjoyment at the table. Eating is more than just about fueling our bodies; it's a social experience, a moment of connection. I've seen people with dysphagia feel left out or embarrassed at family dinners because they couldn't eat the same foods as everyone else. A modified diet changes that. By carefully preparing meals that are both safe and flavorful, people can participate in meals again. They can enjoy food without fear and reconnect with those around them. It brings joy back to an experience that had become stressful.

Moreover, a modified diet improves digestion. When food isn't chewed or swallowed properly, it can cause all sorts of uncomfortable digestive issues. By adapting the texture of food, digestion becomes smoother and more efficient, leading to better absorption of nutrients. This is particularly important for individuals who already struggle with other health conditions and need to ensure their body is functioning as well as possible.

For caregivers, following a modified diet plan brings a sense of relief. I've seen how overwhelming it can be to balance safety with nutrition, especially when you're caring for someone you love. A modified diet provides a clear structure, giving you

confidence that the meals you're preparing

are not only safe but are also providing everything needed to support health and well-being.

A modified diet isn't just about food—it's about quality of life. It's about making sure that no one has to give up the enjoyment of eating, even when swallowing becomes difficult. By taking the time to understand the needs of someone with dysphagia, and by making thoughtful adjustments to meals, we can help them eat confidently and with pleasure again. This diet brings freedom—freedom from the fear of choking, the fear of aspiration, and the fear of missing out. It's a small change that makes a huge difference.

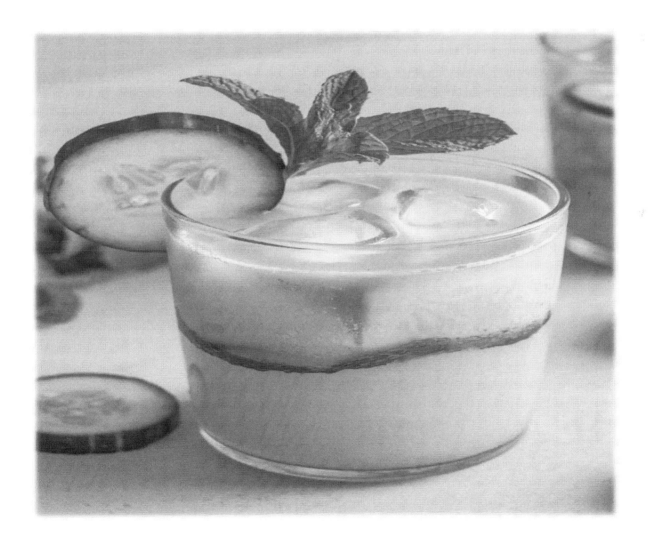

19

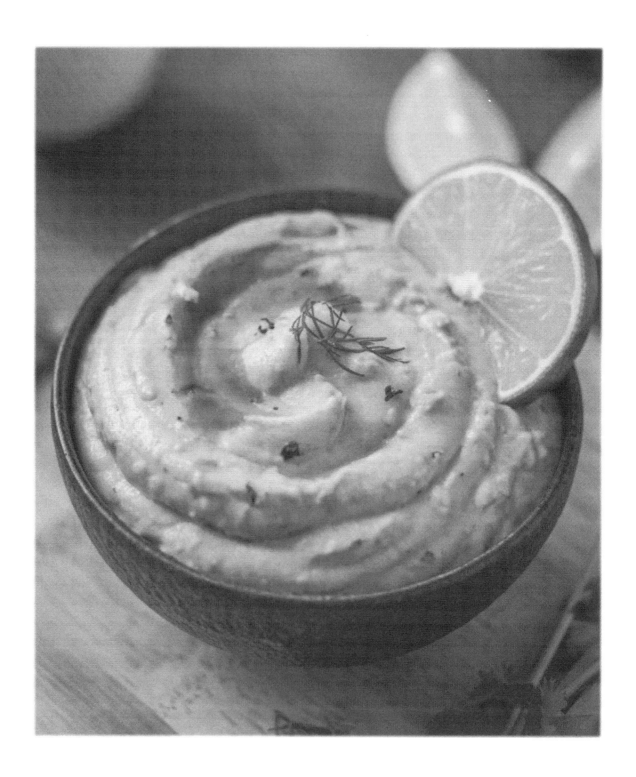

Chapter 2

Overview of Dysphagia Diet Levels

A dysphagia diet is carefully structured to ensure that people with swallowing difficulties can eat safely while still receiving proper nutrition. The diet is divided into levels based on the texture and consistency of food and liquids, designed to reduce the risk of choking or aspiration. Each level corresponds to the individual's ability to safely swallow certain types of foods, and understanding these levels is crucial for managing dysphagia.

The dysphagia diet is generally divided into **three primary levels**, with each level representing a progression in texture as the individual's swallowing ability improves or stabilizes. These levels ensure that food can be swallowed easily and safely, preventing potential complications like aspiration pneumonia, choking, or malnutrition.

Level 1: Pureed Foods (Smooth, No Chewing Required)

This is the most restrictive level of the dysphagia diet, and it's designed for individuals who have significant difficulty swallowing or have little control over their tongue or mouth movements. At this stage, all food must be pureed to a smooth, pudding-like consistency to reduce the risk of aspiration or choking. Foods in this category should be completely free of lumps, chunks, or pieces, ensuring they slide easily down the throat without requiring any chewing. The idea is that the food can be swallowed with minimal effort.

Examples of foods in Level 1 include creamy soups that have been blended, pureed vegetables, mashed potatoes, smooth applesauce, and blended meats. Liquids can also be thickened to a similar consistency to help with swallowing. These pureed foods maintain nutritional value but are modified to ensure that individuals can safely consume them without the risk of food entering the airway. This level is essential for those who may not have the muscle strength or coordination to chew and swallow solid foods.

Level 2: Mechanically Altered/Soft Foods (Some Chewing Required)

Level 2 represents a progression from pureed foods to foods that are soft, moist, and require a little bit of chewing. This level is suitable for individuals who still have difficulty swallowing but have more control over their mouth and throat muscles than those on a Level 1 diet. The texture of the food at this level should be soft enough to easily break apart with a fork and should not contain any large chunks that could pose a choking hazard.

The foods in Level 2 can be mashed, ground, or finely chopped to ensure they can be swallowed easily with minimal effort. While some chewing is required, it is typically light, and the food must still be moist and easy to swallow. Soft-cooked vegetables, ground meats, scrambled eggs, and soft fruits like bananas or peaches are common examples of foods that fit into this category. Casseroles with soft ingredients, well-cooked pasta, and oatmeal are also appropriate, provided they are moist and not sticky.

This level allows for more variety and texture than Level 1, making meals more enjoyable while still being safe. It strikes a balance between offering some texture while ensuring that the food can easily pass through the throat without becoming stuck or triggering choking.

Level 3: Advanced/Soft-Solid Foods (Easy to Chew, Near-Normal)

Level 3 introduces more solid foods that require regular chewing but are still soft and easy to manage. This level is appropriate for individuals who have regained more control over their swallowing muscles but still need to avoid certain foods that could present a choking hazard, such as crunchy, hard, or sticky foods. Level 3 is often used as a transition phase for individuals who are preparing to return to a regular diet, but still need to avoid foods that require a lot of effort to chew or are difficult to swallow.

In this phase, foods should be soft, bite-sized, and easy to chew. Tender cooked meats, soft sandwiches, soft fruits without tough skins (such as ripe peaches or melons), casseroles, and soft bread are suitable for this level. Foods like rice, pasta, and finely chopped salads are allowed, as long as they are soft and not sticky. Items like pancakes, soft muffins, and eggs are typically included, offering a wider range of choices and more normalcy in the diet.

At Level 3, foods are typically moist but not blended or pureed, offering more variety and satisfaction in terms of texture and flavor. However, it's still essential to avoid foods that are hard, crunchy, or require significant chewing, such as nuts, seeds, chips, or raw vegetables.

Understanding these levels and knowing which foods are appropriate for each stage is key to providing a safe and enjoyable eating experience for those with dysphagia.

Texture Modifications for Safe Eating

Texture modification is a fundamental aspect of managing dysphagia, and it plays a crucial role in ensuring that individuals with swallowing difficulties can eat safely. By altering the texture of food and liquids, you can reduce the risk of choking and aspiration, making it easier for those with dysphagia to enjoy their meals without fear. Texture modifications focus on adjusting food to a form that is easier to chew, swallow, and pass through the esophagus without causing complications.

The degree of texture modification required depends on the severity of the individual's swallowing difficulty. While some may only need minor adjustments, such as softening food, others may require foods to be completely pureed. Understanding how to modify textures appropriately is essential for caregivers and individuals alike, as it ensures that meals are both nutritious and safe.

One of the primary modifications is *pureeing food,* which is necessary for individuals with the most severe forms of dysphagia. Pureed foods are completely smooth, free of lumps or chunks, and have a pudding-like consistency. This texture is ideal for those who cannot chew or who have poor control of their tongue and throat muscles. Pureed food can be made from a wide variety of ingredients, including vegetables, fruits, meats, and even starches like potatoes. The key is to blend the food until it is entirely smooth, ensuring it can be swallowed with minimal effort. Adding liquids like broth, milk, or water can help achieve the right consistency without diluting the flavor or nutritional content.

In cases where some **chewing is possible but still limited**, foods can be mechanically altered by mashing, chopping, or finely dicing them. This form of texture modification is suitable for individuals who have difficulty with larger chunks of food but can manage soft, bite-sized pieces. The food should be moist and easily broken apart with a fork. For example, soft-cooked vegetables can be mashed or chopped into small pieces, while meats can be ground or finely shredded. This ensures that the food requires only minimal chewing and won't get stuck in the throat.

Softening food is another common method of texture modification. Certain foods can naturally be made softer through cooking methods like steaming, boiling, or slow cooking. For example, tough meats can be braised or slow-cooked to become tender enough for someone with dysphagia to chew easily. Vegetables can be steamed until they are very soft, and grains like rice or pasta can be cooked until they are tender and moist. Adding sauces or gravies to dishes can also help by adding moisture, making the food easier to swallow without requiring significant effort.

Thickening liquids is another essential part of texture modification. For individuals with dysphagia, thin liquids like water, juice, or broth can easily enter the airway, leading to aspiration. Thickening agents, such as commercial thickeners,

Dysphagia cookbook for beginners

cornstarch, or pureed fruits, can be added to liquids to give them a nectar-like or honey-like consistency, depending on the individual's needs. These thicker liquids move more slowly down the throat, allowing the person more control during swallowing and reducing the risk of the liquid entering the airway.

In addition to thickening liquids, some individuals may benefit from modifying the texture of foods that have mixed consistencies. Foods like soups with both liquid and solid components (e.g., broth with chunks of vegetables or meat) can be particularly challenging for those with dysphagia, as the solids and liquids may be swallowed at different rates, increasing the risk of aspiration. For these types of meals, it's often best to puree the entire dish or ensure that the solid components are soft and well-integrated with the liquid. This way, everything moves down the throat at the same pace, reducing the risk of choking or aspiration.

It's also important to avoid certain textures that pose a higher risk for those with dysphagia. Foods that are sticky, hard, dry, or crumbly can easily become lodged in the throat or airway. Sticky foods, such as peanut butter or thick, gummy candies, tend to adhere to the roof of the mouth or the throat, making them difficult to swallow. Dry foods like crackers or toast, as well as crumbly foods like chips or cookies, can break into small, sharp pieces that are hard to control when swallowing. These textures should either be avoided or heavily modified by adding moisture or breaking them down into safer forms.

Texture modification isn't just about safety; it's also about ensuring that meals remain appealing and nutritious. While it can be challenging to adjust textures, especially for individuals who miss the variety of textures in their meals, it's possible to get creative in the kitchen. By using herbs, spices, and sauces, pureed and soft foods can still be full of flavor. Presentation also matters; even though food may need to be blended or mashed, it can still be plated in a visually appealing way, helping to preserve the dignity and enjoyment of the eating experience.

For those managing dysphagia, texture modification becomes second nature with time. It's an adaptive approach that prioritizes safety without sacrificing the pleasure of a good meal. By making thoughtful changes to the consistency of food and liquids, individuals with dysphagia can continue to enjoy diverse, nutritious meals while minimizing the risks associated with swallowing difficulties.

Essential Ingredients for Every Dysphagia-Friendly Kitchen

A dysphagia-friendly kitchen requires a set of essential ingredients that cater to the modified textures and consistency necessary for safe swallowing while maintaining nutrition and flavor. These ingredients help create meals that are easy to swallow, yet enjoyable and nourishing. Whether you are preparing pureed foods, soft meals, or thickened liquids, having the right staples on hand will ensure that you can make a wide variety of dishes that meet the needs of someone with dysphagia.

One of the most important ingredients in a dysphagia-friendly kitchen is **thickening agents.** These are used to alter the consistency of liquids and some foods, making them safer to swallow. Commercial thickeners are widely available and come in both powder and liquid form, designed specifically for people with dysphagia. They can be added to soups, smoothies, juices, or even water to give them a thicker consistency that is easier to control when swallowing. Cornstarch, tapioca starch, and potato starch can also act as natural thickening agents in home-cooked meals. Additionally, pureed fruits like applesauce or mashed bananas can be used to thicken smoothies or other blended dishes.

Broth and stock are essential in a dysphagia kitchen, especially for adding moisture to meals and ensuring that foods stay soft and easy to swallow. Whether it's chicken, beef, or vegetable broth, these liquids can be added to meats, grains, or vegetables to soften them and make them more palatable. Broth is also a versatile base for soups that can be pureed or made thicker with added ingredients, creating hearty yet manageable dishes.

Full-fat dairy products such as milk, cream, and yogurt are incredibly useful in preparing dysphagia-friendly meals. They not only add moisture but also boost the calorie and nutrient content of meals, which is especially important for individuals who may struggle to eat large portions. Creamy dairy products can be mixed into mashed potatoes, pureed vegetables, or blended with fruits to create smooth, high-calorie meals that are easier to swallow. Yogurt can be served on its own or blended into smoothies for a smooth, thick consistency that provides both protein and calcium.

Nut butters and soft spreads like peanut butter, almond butter, or cream cheese are excellent ingredients to have on hand, but it's important to modify them for safe swallowing. Nut butters can be thinned with liquids like milk or broth to make them less sticky and easier to manage. These spreads provide healthy fats and can be mixed into other dishes or spread on soft breads for added flavor and nutrition. Cream cheese can be used in pureed or softened dishes to add a creamy texture and a rich flavor that elevates simple meals.

Pureed fruits and vegetables are another must-have in a dysphagia-friendly kitchen. Ready-made purees, such as applesauce or baby food, are convenient options, but you can also prepare your own at home using a blender or food processor. Pureed carrots, sweet potatoes, peas, and other vegetables can serve as bases for soups or side dishes. Fruits like bananas, peaches, and pears can be blended into smooth, easy-to-swallow desserts or breakfast options. These purees are rich in vitamins and fiber, ensuring that individuals with dysphagia still get their essential nutrients in a form that's easier to digest.

For added nutrition and variety, soft proteins such as eggs, tofu, and ground meats are key. Scrambled eggs, soft-boiled eggs, and egg custards can be made light and moist, making them ideal for individuals on a dysphagia diet. Tofu is another versatile protein source that can be blended into soups, mashed into soft meals, or used in smoothies for added texture and protein. Ground meats, when cooked until tender and moist, can be blended or finely mashed with sauces or broths to create soft, flavorful dishes that provide essential protein.

Pasta and grains that can be cooked until very soft are also important staples in a dysphagia-friendly kitchen. Overcooked pasta, rice, and quinoa become tender and easy to manage when combined with sauces or pureed vegetables. These grains can serve as a base for many meals, adding bulk and carbohydrates without requiring a lot of chewing. For an even smoother texture, grains can be blended into soups or casseroles, ensuring they are moist enough to swallow comfortably.

Smooth sauces and gravies are another crucial addition to meals for those with dysphagia. Whether you're making a cream sauce, tomato-based sauce, or a simple gravy, these liquids add moisture and flavor to foods, making them easier to swallow. Smooth sauces also help soften proteins like chicken or beef, while gravies can be used to moisten breads or mashed dishes, ensuring that every bite goes down smoothly.

Frozen fruits and vegetables are convenient and versatile ingredients for a dysphagia-friendly kitchen. They can be easily steamed, boiled, or pureed to create smooth textures. Frozen fruits like berries and mangoes can be blended into smoothies, while vegetables like spinach or peas can be added to soups or pureed on their own. These ingredients offer flexibility and ease, making meal prep simpler for caregivers and ensuring that meals are always nutrient-dense.

Substitutes for Common Foods

When managing dysphagia, some common foods need to be avoided or altered to prevent choking or aspiration. Fortunately, there are many substitutes that can replace these foods while still maintaining nutrition, flavor, and safety for individuals with swallowing difficulties. These substitutes help to modify textures without sacrificing taste, allowing people with dysphagia to enjoy a wide variety of meals.

Dysphagia cookbook for beginners

For bread and other dry, crumbly foods that can be difficult to swallow, a good substitute is soft, moist alternatives. Instead of toast or dry crackers, opt for soft pancakes, waffles, or soft rolls soaked in broth, milk, or sauces. These options provide a similar flavor and structure but are easier to swallow. You can also use bread that's softened with gravy, soups, or spreads like softened cream cheese or mashed avocado to create a safer texture.

Instead of **raw vegetables**, which can be hard, fibrous, and difficult to chew, you can use well-cooked, soft vegetables as a substitute. Steaming or boiling vegetables like carrots, zucchini, spinach, or squash until they are very soft ensures that they're easier to chew and swallow. You can also puree these vegetables to achieve a smooth texture. For salads, swap raw greens with cooked spinach or pureed vegetables in a savory dressing.

Tough or chewy meats can be hard to manage for people with dysphagia, so a suitable substitute would be ground, minced, or shredded meats cooked until they're very tender. Ground beef, chicken, turkey, or pork can be cooked in sauces or broths to ensure they stay moist and easy to swallow. Another great alternative is fish, such as baked or poached salmon or tilapia, which tends to be naturally soft and flaky. For a plant-based alternative, tofu is an excellent protein source that's soft, easy to blend, and can be flavored to suit different dishes.

For those who enjoy nuts and seeds, which can be choking hazards, you can use nut butters as a safer substitute. Peanut butter, almond butter, and cashew butter can be thinned with milk or yogurt to make them easier to swallow. Nut butters provide the same healthy fats and protein as whole nuts but are much easier to modify for texture. Another option is blending nuts into smoothies or adding them to purees to ensure they are finely ground.

When it comes to **rice and other dry grains**, which can be difficult to manage because they scatter in the mouth, a good alternative is overcooked grains. Overcooking rice, quinoa, or pasta until they're very soft and moist makes them easier to swallow. You can also puree grains into a porridge-like consistency or mix them with sauces to add moisture and create a smoother texture. Risotto and soft polenta are other great grain-based alternatives that are naturally creamy and easy to swallow.

For **crunchy snacks like chips, crackers, or pretzels,** a safer substitute would be soft snacks such as pudding, applesauce, yogurt, or mashed fruits like bananas or peaches. These alternatives provide similar satisfaction without the risk of dry, crumbly textures getting stuck in the throat. You can also make soft snacks like gelatin or custard, which are safe and enjoyable for individuals with dysphagia.

Fruit with tough skins, such as apples, pears, or grapes, can be substituted with peeled or cooked fruits. You can easily peel and cook apples or pears to soften them, or opt for naturally soft fruits like bananas, ripe peaches, or melons. Pureed fruits are also a great substitute and can be enjoyed as smoothies, blended desserts, or spoonable purees. Canned fruits packed in water or their own juice can also be a softer, easier-to-swallow option.

For hard cheeses, which can be chewy and difficult to break down, soft cheeses such as cream cheese, ricotta, or cottage cheese are great alternatives. These cheeses can be easily mixed into dishes or used as a spread. Soft cheeses have a smooth texture that's easy to swallow and can add creaminess and flavor to many meals. You can also use melted cheese or cheese sauces to incorporate dairy into soft, manageable dishes.

When it comes to **crunchy cereals or granola,** a safer substitute would be cooked cereals such as oatmeal, cream of wheat, or grits. These hot cereals are naturally soft and can be made even smoother by blending them with milk or yogurt. For extra flavor, you can add pureed fruits, cinnamon, or honey. These substitutes provide the same satisfying warmth as traditional cereals but in a safer form for swallowing.

By using these substitutes, individuals with dysphagia can still enjoy many of their favorite foods, with the peace of mind that each meal will be safe and satisfying. These modifications help maintain variety and nutrition while ensuring that textures are manageable for those with swallowing difficulties.

Special Thickening Agents and Their Uses

Special thickening agents play a crucial role in preparing food and beverages for individuals with dysphagia. These agents modify the consistency of liquids and some foods, making them easier to swallow and reducing the risk of aspiration, choking, or food entering the airway. The right thickening agent can transform thin, runny liquids into thicker, more manageable consistencies that move more slowly through the throat, giving individuals with dysphagia better control during swallowing. Each type of thickening agent has unique properties and uses, making it important to choose the right one depending on the food or beverage being prepared.

One of the most widely used thickening agents in a dysphagia diet is **commercial thickeners.** These are specially formulated products designed to modify the consistency of both hot and cold liquids. Commercial thickeners typically come in two forms: powder and gel. They are easy to use and have been developed to provide predictable results, allowing for the precise control of the liquid's consistency. Depending on how much thickener is used, liquids can be thickened to different levels, such as nectar-like, honey-like, or spoon-thick. Many commercial thickeners are flavorless and dissolve easily, making them ideal for beverages like water, juice, tea, or coffee. Some popular brands of commercial thickeners include Thick-It and SimplyThick.

Cornstarch is another thickening agent that can be used in home-cooked meals. It's a versatile, pantry staple that thickens liquids quickly when heated. Cornstarch is especially useful in making gravies, soups, or sauces for individuals with dysphagia. When mixed with water or broth, cornstarch can help create a smooth, thick consistency that's easy to swallow. However, cornstarch can alter the flavor of certain liquids and is not always ideal for cold drinks. It works best for cooked dishes

31

that require some heat to activate the thickening properties.

Potato starch is another naturally occurring thickener that works similarly to cornstarch. It is often used in soups, stews, and sauces to create a creamy, thick consistency. Potato starch can also be added to blended or pureed foods to give them more body without significantly altering the taste. Like cornstarch, it is most effective when used in hot dishes and provides a smooth, lump-free texture when mixed properly.

Tapioca starch is another excellent thickening agent that is derived from the cassava plant. It is particularly useful in both hot and cold dishes and is often used to thicken soups, gravies, and fruit fillings for pies or desserts. Tapioca starch has a slightly different texture from cornstarch, giving food a silky, almost gel-like consistency. It's a great option for individuals with dysphagia who prefer smoother, more fluid textures in their food. Tapioca pearls, a form of tapioca starch, can also be cooked down and pureed to create thick, pudding-like desserts.

For those who prefer more natural thickening agents, pureed fruits can be an effective way to thicken liquids and add nutritional value. Fruits like bananas, avocados, apples, and peaches can be blended into drinks or smoothies to give them a thicker consistency. Pureed fruits can also be used in desserts or added to porridge, yogurt, or cereal to make them easier to swallow. Besides providing the desired texture, pureed fruits also add natural sweetness, fiber, and vitamins, making them a healthy thickening option for individuals with dysphagia.

Gelatin is another thickening agent used in dysphagia diets, particularly for thickening liquids into spoon-thick or soft, gel-like consistencies. Gelatin is commonly used in making jellies, desserts, or thickened beverages that can be scooped with a spoon. It's ideal for individuals who need thicker, more stable consistencies for swallowing. While gelatin requires heat to dissolve and set properly, it creates a firm texture that holds its shape and is easy to consume. However, it may not be suitable for all liquids and can alter the flavor of some beverages.

When thickening liquids, it's important to adjust the consistency based on the individual's needs. Nectar-like consistency is often the first step for individuals who have mild dysphagia. At this stage, liquids flow like fruit nectars and are slightly thicker than water, making them easier to control during swallowing. Honey-like consistency is thicker than nectar and flows more slowly, resembling the texture of honey. This consistency provides even more control, making it ideal for individuals who struggle with thin liquids. Spoon-thick liquids have the highest level of thickness, resembling the consistency of pudding or custard. These are eaten with a spoon and are often recommended for individuals with more severe swallowing difficulties.

Dysphagia-Friendly Grocery Guide

Vegetables:
- ✓ Pureed or mashed vegetables (pre-packaged or homemade)
- ✓ Soft-cooked vegetables (carrots, zucchini, spinach, potatoes)
- ✓ Frozen vegetables (peas, spinach, carrots)
- ✓ Canned vegetables (low-sodium green beans, carrots, peas)

Fruits:
- ✓ Pureed fruits (pre-packaged pureed peaches, applesauce)
- ✓ Soft, ripe fruits (bananas, avocados, peaches, melons)
- ✓ Canned fruits (in juice: peaches, pears, fruit cocktail)
- ✓ Frozen fruits (berries, mangoes, peaches)

Proteins:
- ✓ Ground meats (ground chicken, turkey, beef, pork)

- ✓ Soft fish (salmon, tilapia, cod, canned tuna/salmon)
- ✓ Soft proteins (scrambled eggs, soft-boiled eggs, tofu)
- ✓ Blended or pureed meats (pre-packaged or homemade with broth)
- ✓ Beans and lentils (canned, easily mashed or pureed)

Dairy:
- ✓ Smooth dairy products (yogurt without chunks, cottage cheese, ricotta cheese, cream cheese)
- ✓ Milk and alternatives (regular or lactose-free milk, almond milk, oat milk)
- ✓ Soft cheeses (mozzarella, Brie, soft spreadable cheeses)

Grains and Breads:
- ✓ Cooked cereals (cream of wheat, oatmeal, grits, polenta)
- ✓ Soft pasta (cooked until soft, served with sauces)
- ✓ Soft breads (soft sandwich bread, pancakes, waffles, soft rolls)
- ✓ Rice and grains (overcooked rice, couscous, quinoa)

Soups and Liquids:
- ✓ Smooth, pureed soups (cream of tomato, butternut squash, blended chicken soup)
- ✓ Broths and stocks (chicken, beef, vegetable broths)
- ✓ Thickened liquids (commercially thickened beverages or thickened with powders/gels)

Condiments and Sauces:
- ✓ Smooth sauces (gravy, smooth tomato sauce, cheese sauce, hollandaise)
- ✓ Pureed spreads (hummus, mashed avocado, thinned nut butters)

Thickening Agents:
- ✓ Commercial thickeners (Thick-It, SimplyThick)
- ✓ Natural thickeners (cornstarch, potato starch, tapioca starch, xanthan gum)
- ✓ Pureed fruits/vegetables (mashed bananas, avocados, pureed apples/squash)

Chapter 3

Level 1: Pureed Foods (Smooth, No Chewing Required)

Puréed Mango Coconut Rice Pudding

Prep Time: 15 mins | Cook Time: 30 mins | Serves: 4
Per Serving: Calories: 230 | Fat: 8g | Carbs: 35g | Fiber: 2g | Protein: 4g

Ingredients

- 1 cup cooked rice
- 1/2 cup coconut milk
- 1/2 cup fresh mango, diced
- 2 tbsp honey (optional)
- 1/2 tsp vanilla extract

Procedure

1. If you don't have already cooked rice, cook 1 cup of rice according to package instructions (about 2 cups water to 1 cup rice). Allow the rice to cool.

2. In a blender, combine the cooled rice and coconut milk. Blend for 1-2 minutes until smooth.The mixture should be creamy without any lumps.

3. Add the diced mango, honey (if using), and vanilla extract to the blender. Blend again until all ingredients are fully incorporated and the pudding is smooth.

4. Pour the rice pudding into small serving bowls and refrigerate for at least 30 minutes to let the flavors meld together.

5. You can garnish with additional pureed mango or coconut flakes for extra flavor. Serve chilled.

Creamy Oatmeal

(Blended for Smooth Texture)

Prep Time: 5 mins | Cook Time: 10 mins | Serves: 4

Per Serving: Calories: 180 | Fat: 4g | Carbs: 30g | Fiber: 4g | Protein: 6g

Ingredients

- 1 cup rolled oats

- 2 cups milk or milk alternative

- 1 tbsp honey or maple syrup (optional)

- 1/2 tsp cinnamon

Procedure

1. Cook the oats: In a small saucepan, combine 1 cup of rolled oats and 2 cups of milk (or your preferred milk alternative). Place the saucepan over medium heat. Stir occasionally to prevent the oats from sticking to the bottom of the pan. Cook for about 5-7 minutes, until the oats are soft and the mixture thickens.

2. Blend the oatmeal: Once the oats are cooked, transfer the mixture to a blender while it's still hot. Blend for 1-2 minutes until the oatmeal is completely smooth and creamy. Be careful of steam; you may need to leave the lid slightly open to allow it to escape.

3. Add flavorings: Add honey or maple syrup for sweetness, and sprinkle in the cinnamon. Blend again briefly to incorporate these ingredients.

4. Pour the creamy oatmeal into bowls and serve warm. If it thickens too much as it cools, you can stir in a little extra milk before serving.

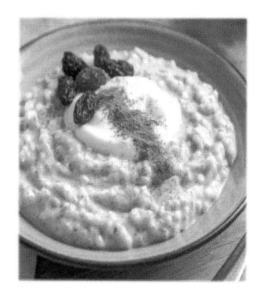

Puréed Fruit Smoothie

Prep Time: 5 mins | Cook Time: 0 mins | Serves: 2

Per Serving: Calories: 150 | Fat: 2g | Carbs: 32g | Fiber: 5g | Protein: 3g

Ingredients

- 1 banana
- 1/2 cup frozen berries
- 1/2 cup Greek yogurt
- 1/2 cup milk or almond milk
- 1 tbsp honey (optional)

Procedure

1. Prepare the ingredients: Peel the banana and break it into smaller pieces. Measure out 1/2 cup of frozen berries (such as strawberries, blueberries, or raspberries).

2. Blend the ingredients: In a blender, add the banana pieces, frozen berries, Greek yogurt, and milk. Blend for 1-2 minutes, until the mixture is completely smooth and thick.

3. Adjust the consistency: If the smoothie is too thick, add a little more milk (a tablespoon at a time) and blend until it reaches the desired consistency.

4. Taste and sweeten: Taste the smoothie and, if you prefer it sweeter, add 1 tablespoon of honey and blend again.

5. Pour the smoothie into glasses and serve immediately. This is a refreshing and nutritious option for breakfast.

Dysphagia cookbook for beginners

Creamy Banana and Peanut Butter Oatmeal

Prep Time: 5 mins | Cook Time: 10 mins | Serves: 4

Per Serving: Calories: 250 | Fat: 10g | Carbs: 32g | Fiber: 4g | Protein: 7g

Ingredients

- 1 cup rolled oats
- 2 cups milk or milk alternative
- 1 banana, mashed
- 2 tbsp smooth peanut butter
- 1 tbsp honey (optional)

Procedure

1. Cook the oats: In a medium saucepan, combine the rolled oats and milk. Cook over medium heat, stirring occasionally, for about 5-7 minutes until the oats are soft and the mixture thickens.

2. Prepare the banana: While the oats are cooking, peel and mash the banana in a small bowl using a fork.

3. Blend the oatmeal: Once the oats are fully cooked, pour the oatmeal into a blender. Add the mashed banana and smooth peanut butter. Blend on medium speed until the mixture is completely smooth and creamy.

4. If desired, add 1 tablespoon of honey for extra sweetness, and blend again. Serve the oatmeal warm. If it becomes too thick as it cools, stir in a little more milk to loosen the texture.

Lemon Ricotta Pancake Purée

Prep Time: 10 mins | Cook Time: 15 mins | Serves: 4
Per Serving: Calories: 210 | Fat: 9g | Carbs: 22g | Fiber: 1g | Protein: 8g

Ingredients

- 1/2 cup ricotta cheese
- 1/2 cup milk
- 1 tbsp lemon juice
- 1 tsp lemon zest
- 2 tbsp honey or sugar
- 1/2 cup cooked soft pancakes

Procedure

1. If you don't have soft pancakes prepared, cook a small batch according to your favorite recipe or use pre-made pancakes. Once cooked, allow them to cool slightly.

2. In a blender, combine the ricotta cheese, milk, lemon juice, lemon zest, and honey (or sugar). Blend on high speed for about 1 minute, until the mixture is smooth and creamy.

3. Tear the cooked pancakes into small bite-sized pieces and add them to the blender. Blend for an additional 1-2 minutes until the pancakes are fully incorporated and the mixture has a smooth, thick consistency.

4. If the purée is too thick, add a little more milk (1 tablespoon at a time) and blend until it reaches your desired consistency.

5. Pour the purée into bowls and serve warm or chilled, depending on your preference.

Savory Tomato Basil Omelette Purée

Prep Time: 10 mins | Cook Time: 10 mins | Serves: 2

Per Serving: Calories: 150 | Fat: 10g | Carbs: 5g | Fiber: 1g | Protein: 8g

Ingredients

- 2 eggs
- 1/4 cup milk
- 1 small tomato, finely chopped
- 2 basil leaves, chopped
- 1 tbsp butter
- Salt and pepper to taste

Procedure

1. Cook the omelette: Crack the eggs into a bowl, add the milk, and whisk until smooth. In a non-stick skillet, melt the butter over medium heat. Add the egg mixture and cook slowly, stirring occasionally to prevent browning. Once the eggs are mostly set, sprinkle the chopped tomato and basil on top. Continue cooking for 1-2 minutes until the eggs are fully cooked and the tomatoes have softened.

2. Transfer to blender: Remove the omelette from the pan and transfer it to a blender. Add 2-3 tablespoons of water or broth to help with blending.

3. Blend until smooth: Blend on medium speed for 1-2 minutes until the omelette is fully pureed and smooth.

4. Add salt and pepper to taste, and blend again briefly. Serve warm.

Pureed Sweet Potato Mash

(with a Touch of Cinnamon)

Prep Time: 10 mins | Cook Time: 20 mins | Serves: 4
Per Serving: Calories: 180 | Fat: 3g | Carbs: 35g | Fiber: 4g | Protein: 3g

Ingredients

- 2 large sweet potatoes, peeled and chopped
- 1/4 cup milk
- 1 tbsp butter
- 1 tsp cinnamon
- 1 tbsp honey (optional)

Procedure

1. Boil the sweet potatoes: In a medium pot, bring water to a boil. Add the peeled and chopped sweet potatoes and cook for 15-20 minutes, until they are soft and can be easily pierced with a fork. Drain the water.

2. Blend the sweet potatoes: Transfer the cooked sweet potatoes to a blender or food processor. Add the milk, butter, and cinnamon. Blend for 1-2 minutes until the mixture is smooth and creamy.

3. Adjust sweetness: If you prefer a sweeter mash, add honey and blend again to incorporate.

4. Serve warm as a comforting and flavorful side dish.

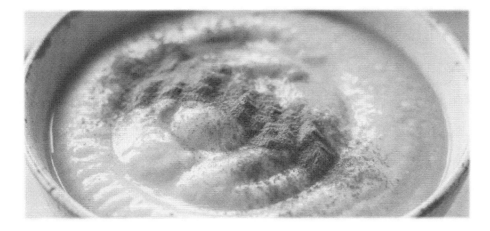

41

Puréed Avocado Toast

(Blended Avocado with Pureed Bread)

Prep Time: 5 mins | Cook Time: 0 mins | Serves: 2

Per Serving: Calories: 220 | Fat: 16g | Carbs: 20g | Fiber: 6g | Protein: 4g

Ingredients

- 1 ripe avocado
- 2 slices soft sandwich bread
- 1 tbsp lemon juice
- Salt and pepper to taste
- Optional: 1 tbsp olive oil for extra creaminess

Procedure

1. Prepare the avocado: Slice the avocado in half, remove the pit, and scoop the flesh into a blender. Add the lemon juice to keep it fresh and add a bit of tang.

2. Puree the bread: Tear the soft sandwich bread into small pieces and add it to the blender with the avocado. Optionally, add 1 tablespoon of olive oil for extra smoothness.

3. Blend until smooth: Blend the mixture for 1-2 minutes until the bread and avocado are fully combined and smooth.

4. Season with salt and pepper, blend briefly, and serve immediately. This smooth puree is a great way to enjoy the flavors of avocado toast without the chewing.

Dysphagia cookbook for beginners

Peaches and Cream Purée

Prep Time: 5 mins | Cook Time: 0 mins | Serves: 2

Per Serving: Calories: 140 | Fat: 6g | Carbs: 20g | Fiber: 2g | Protein: 3g

Ingredients

- 1 cup canned peaches (in juice, drained)
- 1/4 cup heavy cream or yogurt
- 1 tbsp honey (optional)

Procedure

1. Prepare the peaches: Drain the canned peaches, ensuring there is no excess liquid, and add them to a blender.

2. Add cream: Pour in the heavy cream or yogurt to add smoothness and richness to the puree.

3. Blend until smooth: Blend for 1-2 minutes until the peaches and cream are fully combined and smooth.

4. Taste and sweeten: If desired, add honey for extra sweetness and blend again.

5. Pour into serving bowls and refrigerate for a few minutes before serving, or enjoy immediately.

Quick Lunch

Puréed Chicken and Vegetable Soup

Prep Time: 10 mins | Cook Time: 30 mins | Serves: 4
Per Serving: Calories: 180 | Fat: 5g | Carbs: 20g | Fiber: 3g | Protein: 15g

Ingredients

- 1 lb boneless, skinless chicken breast
- 2 carrots, peeled and chopped
- 1 small potato, peeled and chopped
- 1 celery stalk, chopped
- 1 small onion, chopped
- 4 cups low-sodium chicken broth
- 1/4 tsp thyme (optional)
- Salt and pepper to taste

Procedure

1. Cook the chicken and vegetables: In a large pot, combine the chicken, chopped carrots, potato, celery, onion, and chicken broth. Bring the mixture to a boil over medium heat, then reduce the heat to low and let it simmer for about 20 minutes, until the chicken is fully cooked and the vegetables are tender.

2. Remove the chicken: Once the chicken is cooked, remove it from the pot and set it aside for a moment.

3. Blend the vegetables: Transfer the vegetables and broth to a blender. Blend on high until the mixture is smooth and creamy.

4. Shred and puree the chicken: Cut the chicken into smaller pieces and add it to the blender with the pureed vegetables. Blend for another 1-2 minutes until the chicken is fully incorporated and the soup has a smooth consistency.

5. Add thyme, salt, and pepper to taste, and blend briefly to mix. Serve the soup warm.

Creamy Mashed Potatoes with Soft Meatloaf Purée

Prep Time: 15 mins | Cook Time: 30 mins | Serves: 4

Per Serving: Calories: 320 | Fat: 15g | Carbs: 30g | Fiber: 4g | Protein: 20g

Ingredients

- 4 medium potatoes, peeled and chopped
- 1/4 cup milk
- 2 tbsp butter
- 1 lb ground beef or turkey
- 1/4 cup breadcrumbs
- 1 egg
- 1/4 cup ketchup
- 1/2 tsp salt
- 1/4 tsp pepper

Procedure

1. Prepare the meatloaf: Preheat your oven to 350°F (175°C). In a mixing bowl, combine the ground beef (or turkey), breadcrumbs, egg, ketchup, salt, and pepper. Mix well until all ingredients are combined. Press the mixture into a loaf pan and bake for about 30 minutes, or until the meatloaf is fully cooked.

2. Boil the potatoes: While the meatloaf is baking, bring a pot of water to a boil. Add the chopped potatoes and cook for about 15-20 minutes until they are soft and easily pierced with a fork. Drain the water.

3. Mash the potatoes: In a blender, combine the cooked potatoes, milk, and butter. Blend until smooth and creamy.

4. Puree the meatloaf: Once the meatloaf is cooked, cut it into smaller pieces and transfer it to the blender. Add a small amount of broth or water to help blend. Blend on medium speed for 1-2 minutes until the meatloaf reaches a smooth consistency.

5. Serve the pureed meatloaf alongside the creamy mashed potatoes. You can blend them together or serve them separately.

Puréed Spinach and Ricotta Lasagna

Prep Time: 15 mins | Cook Time: 40 mins | Serves: 4

Per Serving: Calories: 290 | Fat: 12g | Carbs: 25g | Fiber: 3g | Protein: 18g

Ingredients

- 6 lasagna noodles, cooked until soft

- 1 cup ricotta cheese

- 1/2 cup spinach, cooked and drained

- 1/2 cup marinara sauce (smooth, without chunks)

- 1/4 cup mozzarella cheese, shredded

- 1/4 tsp garlic powder

- Salt and pepper to taste

Procedure

1. Cook the lasagna noodles: In a large pot of boiling water, cook the lasagna noodles until very soft (beyond al dente). Drain and set aside.

2. Prepare the spinach ricotta filling: In a small bowl, mix together the ricotta cheese, cooked spinach, garlic powder, salt, and pepper.

3. Layer and bake: In a blender, combine the cooked lasagna noodles, ricotta spinach mixture, and marinara sauce. Blend until smooth, making sure the mixture is well-combined and lump-free.

4. Add cheese: Stir in the shredded mozzarella cheese by hand or blend it into the puree for added creaminess.

5. Bake: Pour the pureed mixture into a greased baking dish and bake at 350°F (175°C) for 20 minutes, or until heated through.

6. Serve warm, garnished with a small drizzle of extra marinara sauce if desired.

Puréed Macaroni and Cheese

Prep Time: 10 mins | Cook Time: 15 mins | Serves: 4

Per Serving: Calories: 250 | Fat: 10g | Carbs: 30g | Fiber: 2g | Protein: 9g

Ingredients

- 2 cups macaroni noodles
- 1/2 cup cheddar cheese, shredded
- 1/4 cup milk
- 1 tbsp butter
- Salt and pepper to taste

Procedure

1. Cook the macaroni: Bring a large pot of water to a boil. Add the macaroni noodles and cook until very soft (beyond al dente). Drain and set aside.

2. Prepare the cheese sauce: In a small saucepan, melt the butter over medium heat. Add the milk and shredded cheddar cheese, stirring continuously until the cheese is fully melted and the sauce is smooth.

3. Puree the macaroni: Transfer the cooked macaroni to a blender. Pour the cheese sauce over the noodles. Blend on medium speed for 1-2 minutes until smooth and creamy.

4. Adjust the consistency: If the mixture is too thick, add a little more milk (1 tbsp at a time) and blend until you reach your desired consistency.

5. Add salt and pepper to taste, and blend briefly to incorporate. Serve warm.

Dysphagia cookbook for beginners

Puréed Vegetable Medley with Soft-Cooked Lentils

Prep Time: 10 mins | Cook Time: 30 mins | Serves: 4
Per Serving: Calories: 220 | Fat: 5g | Carbs: 38g | Fiber: 8g | Protein: 10g

Ingredients

- 1/2 cup dried lentils
- 1 cup carrots, peeled and chopped
- 1 cup zucchini, chopped
- 1/2 cup spinach leaves
- 1/2 cup low-sodium vegetable broth
- 1 tbsp olive oil
- Salt and pepper to taste

Procedure

1. Cook the lentils: Rinse the lentils under cold water. In a medium pot, bring 2 cups of water to a boil, add the lentils, and simmer on low heat for about 20-25 minutes, until the lentils are soft and tender. Drain excess water.

2. Cook the vegetables: In a separate pot, add the carrots, zucchini, spinach, and vegetable broth. Bring to a simmer and cook for 15-20 minutes, or until all the vegetables are tender.

3. Blend the vegetables and lentils: Once the lentils and vegetables are cooked, transfer both to a blender. Add the olive oil and blend until smooth, about 1-2 minutes.

4. Adjust the consistency: If the mixture is too thick, add more broth, 1 tablespoon at a time, until you reach a smooth, pureed consistency.

5. Season with salt and pepper to taste and serve warm.

Puréed Beef Stew with Root Vegetables

Prep Time: 15 mins | Cook Time: 1 hr | Serves: 4

Per Serving: Calories: 350 | Fat: 12g | Carbs: 35g | Fiber: 6g | Protein: 25g

Ingredients

- 1 lb beef stew meat, cut into small cubes
- 2 carrots, peeled and chopped
- 2 potatoes, peeled and chopped
- 1 small onion, chopped
- 2 cups low-sodium beef broth
- 1 tsp thyme
- Salt and pepper to taste

Procedure

1. Cook the beef: In a large pot, add the beef stew meat and cook over medium heat until browned on all sides (about 5-7 minutes).

2. Add vegetables and broth: Add the carrots, potatoes, onion, beef broth, and thyme to the pot. Bring to a boil, then reduce the heat to low and simmer for about 45 minutes, or until the beef is tender and the vegetables are soft.

3. Blend the stew: Remove the stew from heat and allow it to cool slightly. Transfer the entire mixture (meat, vegetables, and broth) to a blender. Blend on high for 2-3 minutes until smooth and creamy.

4. Adjust consistency: If the stew is too thick, add additional broth to achieve a smooth consistency.

5. Add salt and pepper to taste. Serve warm.

Butternut Squash and Apple Purée

Prep Time: 10 mins | Cook Time: 25 mins | Serves: 4
Per Serving: Calories: 160 | Fat: 4g | Carbs: 30g | Fiber: 5g | Protein: 2g

Ingredients

- 2 cups butternut squash, peeled and chopped
- 1 large apple, peeled and chopped
- 1/2 tsp cinnamon
- 1/4 cup water or low-sodium vegetable broth
- 1 tbsp butter

Procedure

1. Cook the squash and apple: In a medium saucepan, combine the butternut squash, apple, and water or broth. Bring to a boil, then reduce heat and simmer for about 20 minutes, or until both the squash and apple are soft.

2. Blend the mixture: Once cooked, transfer the squash and apple to a blender. Add the butter and cinnamon. Blend for 1-2 minutes until smooth and creamy.

3. Adjust consistency: If the puree is too thick, add more water or broth to achieve your desired consistency.

4. Serve warm or chilled, depending on your preference.

Dysphagia cookbook for beginners

Puréed Roasted Red Pepper, Feta, and Chickpeas

Prep Time: 15 mins | Cook Time: 30 mins | Serves: 4

Per Serving: Calories: 210 | Fat: 10g | Carbs: 25g | Fiber: 6g | Protein: 8g

Ingredients

- 2 large red bell peppers, roasted
- 1/2 cup canned chickpeas, rinsed and drained
- 1/4 cup feta cheese, crumbled
- 1 tbsp olive oil
- 1/4 cup low-sodium vegetable broth
- Salt and pepper to taste

Procedure

1. Roast the red peppers: Preheat your oven to 400°F (200°C). Place the whole red bell peppers on a baking sheet and roast for 20-30 minutes, turning occasionally, until the skin is charred. Remove from the oven, cool slightly, and peel the skin off.

2. Combine ingredients in the blender: In a blender, add the roasted red peppers, chickpeas, feta cheese, olive oil, and vegetable broth.

3. Blend until smooth: Blend for 1-2 minutes until the mixture is smooth and creamy.

4. Adjust consistency: If needed, add more broth to thin the puree to the desired consistency.

5. Add salt and pepper to taste. Serve warm or chilled.

51

Creamy Celery Root, White Beans, and Apple Soup

Prep Time: 15 mins | Cook Time: 30 mins | Serves: 4

Per Serving: Calories: 190 | Fat: 5g | Carbs: 30g | Fiber: 7g | Protein: 8g

Ingredients

- 2 cups celery root, peeled and chopped
- 1 apple, peeled and chopped
- 1/2 cup white beans (canned, drained, and rinsed)
- 2 cups low-sodium vegetable broth
- 1 tbsp olive oil
- Salt and pepper to taste

Procedure

1. Cook the celery root and apple: In a medium pot, combine the celery root, apple, and vegetable broth. Bring to a boil, then reduce the heat and simmer for 20-25 minutes, or until the celery root and apple are tender.

2. Add the white beans: Add the drained white beans to the pot and cook for an additional 5 minutes.

3. Blend the soup: Transfer the entire mixture to a blender. Add the olive oil and blend for 1-2 minutes until smooth and creamy.

4. Add salt and pepper to taste, and blend briefly to mix. Serve warm.

Tasty Dinner

Carrot and Ginger Soup with Puréed Chicken

Prep Time: 10 mins | Cook Time: 30 mins | Serves: 4
Per Serving: Calories: 230 | Fat: 7g | Carbs: 30g | Fiber: 6g | Protein: 15g

Ingredients

- 1 lb boneless, skinless chicken breast
- 4 large carrots, peeled and chopped
- 1 small onion, chopped
- 1 tbsp fresh ginger, grated
- 4 cups low-sodium chicken broth
- 1 tbsp olive oil
- Salt and pepper to taste

Procedure

1. Cook the chicken: In a pot, bring water to a boil and add the chicken breast. Simmer for 15 minutes, or until fully cooked. Remove and let cool slightly.

2. Prepare the soup: In another pot, heat the olive oil over medium heat. Add the onion, carrots, and ginger, sautéing for 5 minutes.

3. Simmer the vegetables: Add the chicken broth and bring to a boil. Lower the heat and simmer for 20 minutes, until the carrots are soft.

4. Blend the vegetables: Remove from heat and transfer the carrot mixture to a blender. Blend until smooth.

5. Purée the chicken: Add the cooked chicken to the blender with the pureed soup and blend until smooth.

6. Add salt and pepper to taste, blend briefly, and serve warm.

Herbed Puréed Zucchini with Grated Halloumi

Prep Time: 10 mins | Cook Time: 15 mins | Serves: 4

Per Serving: Calories: 200 | Fat: 12g | Carbs: 10g | Fiber: 3g | Protein: 12g

Ingredients

- 4 medium zucchinis, chopped
- 1/4 cup low-sodium vegetable broth
- 1/2 cup halloumi cheese, grated
- 1 tbsp olive oil
- 1/2 tsp dried oregano
- Salt and pepper to taste

Procedure

1. Cook the zucchini: In a medium saucepan, heat the olive oil over medium heat. Add the chopped zucchini and sauté for 5 minutes.

2. Simmer the zucchini: Add the vegetable broth, cover, and cook for another 10 minutes, or until the zucchini is soft.

3. Blend the zucchini: Transfer the cooked zucchini to a blender, add the oregano, and blend until smooth.

4. Incorporate the cheese: Stir in the grated halloumi to add flavor and creaminess.

5. Add salt and pepper to taste, blend briefly, and serve warm.

Puréed Meatloaf with Pureed Carrots

Prep Time: 15 mins | Cook Time: 40 mins | Serves: 4
Per Serving: Calories: 290 | Fat: 15g | Carbs: 25g | Fiber: 4g | Protein: 20g

Ingredients

- 1 lb ground beef or turkey
- 1/4 cup breadcrumbs
- 1 egg
- 1/4 cup ketchup
- 4 large carrots, peeled and chopped
- 1/4 cup milk
- 1 tbsp butter
- Salt and pepper to taste

Procedure

1. Prepare the meatloaf: In a mixing bowl, combine the ground meat, breadcrumbs, egg, and ketchup. Press the mixture into a loaf pan and bake at 350°F (175°C) for 35-40 minutes, or until fully cooked.

2. Cook the carrots: While the meatloaf is cooking, bring a pot of water to a boil and add the chopped carrots. Boil for 15-20 minutes until soft. Drain the water.

3. Purée the carrots: Transfer the cooked carrots to a blender with milk and butter. Blend until smooth and creamy.

4. Purée the meatloaf: Once the meatloaf is fully cooked, cut it into smaller pieces and blend with a little broth or water to achieve a smooth consistency.

5. Serve the puréed meatloaf with the creamy puréed carrots.

Spaghetti Bolognese Puréed

Prep Time: 15 mins | Cook Time: 30 mins | Serves: 4

Per Serving: Calories: 350 | Fat: 15g | Carbs: 40g | Fiber: 5g | Protein: 18g

Ingredients

- 1 lb ground beef or turkey
- 1 small onion, chopped
- 1 cup marinara sauce (smooth, no chunks)
- 6 oz spaghetti, cooked very soft
- 1/2 cup grated Parmesan cheese
- 1/4 cup water or broth
- 1 tbsp olive oil
- Salt and pepper to taste

Procedure

1. Cook the ground meat: In a skillet, heat olive oil over medium heat. Add the chopped onion and ground meat. Cook for 8-10 minutes, until the meat is browned and fully cooked.

2. Add the sauce: Pour in the marinara sauce and simmer for an additional 10 minutes.

3. Cook the spaghetti: Meanwhile, cook the spaghetti in boiling water until very soft (beyond al dente). Drain.

4. Blend the spaghetti and sauce: Transfer the spaghetti and meat sauce to a blender. Add the grated Parmesan cheese and a little water or broth to help achieve a smooth consistency. Blend until fully puréed.

5. Add salt and pepper to taste, blend briefly, and serve warm.

Dysphagia cookbook for beginners

Puréed Chicken Alfredo with Pureed Broccoli

Prep Time: 15 mins | Cook Time: 25 mins | Serves: 4

Per Serving: Calories: 400 | Fat: 20g | Carbs: 25g | Fiber: 4g | Protein: 28g

Ingredients

- 1 lb boneless, skinless chicken breast
- 1 cup heavy cream
- 1/2 cup Parmesan cheese, grated
- 6 oz fettuccine, cooked very soft
- 1 cup broccoli, chopped
- 1 tbsp butter
- Salt and pepper to taste

Procedure

1. Cook the chicken: In a pot, bring water to a boil and add the chicken breast. Simmer for 15 minutes until fully cooked. Remove and set aside.

2. Prepare the Alfredo sauce: In a small saucepan, heat the heavy cream and Parmesan cheese over low heat, stirring until the cheese melts and the sauce thickens slightly.

3. Cook the broccoli: Boil the chopped broccoli in water for 10 minutes, until soft. Drain the water.

4. Purée the chicken and pasta: Blend the cooked chicken, soft fettuccine, and Alfredo sauce until smooth.

5. Purée the broccoli: Blend the broccoli with butter until smooth.

6. Serve the puréed chicken Alfredo with puréed broccoli.

Pumpkin and Apple Soup

Prep Time: 10 mins | Cook Time: 20 mins | Serves: 4

Per Serving: Calories: 180 | Fat: 6g | Carbs: 28g | Fiber: 5g | Protein: 2g

Ingredients

- 2 cups pumpkin purée (canned or cooked)
- 1 large apple, peeled and chopped
- 1 small onion, chopped
- 2 cups low-sodium vegetable broth
- 1/4 tsp cinnamon
- 1/4 tsp nutmeg
- 1 tbsp olive oil
- Salt and pepper to taste

Procedure

1. Cook the apple and onion: In a large saucepan, heat the olive oil over medium heat. Add the chopped apple and onion, sautéing for 5 minutes until softened.

2. Add the pumpkin: Add the pumpkin purée, vegetable broth, cinnamon, and nutmeg. Bring to a boil, then reduce heat and simmer for 15 minutes.

3. Blend the soup: Transfer the mixture to a blender and blend for 1-2 minutes until smooth.

4. Add salt and pepper to taste. Serve warm, garnished with a sprinkle of cinnamon.

Puréed Spicy Tomato and Red Lentil Soup

Prep Time: 10 mins | Cook Time: 30 mins | Serves: 4
Per Serving: Calories: 220 | Fat: 5g | Carbs: 35g | Fiber: 8g | Protein: 10g

Ingredients

- 1 cup red lentils, rinsed
- 1 can (14 oz) diced tomatoes (low-sodium)
- 1 small onion, chopped
- 1 garlic clove, minced
- 1/2 tsp cumin
- 1/4 tsp red pepper flakes (optional)
- 4 cups low-sodium vegetable broth
- 1 tbsp olive oil
- Salt and pepper to taste

Procedure

1. Cook the lentils: In a medium saucepan, combine the red lentils and vegetable broth. Bring to a boil, then reduce heat and simmer for 15-20 minutes until the lentils are soft.

2. Sauté the vegetables: In a skillet, heat olive oil and sauté the chopped onion and garlic for 5 minutes until soft.

3. Combine and simmer: Add the canned tomatoes, cumin, and red pepper flakes to the skillet and cook for 5 more minutes.

4. Blend the soup: Transfer the lentils and vegetable mixture to a blender. Blend for 1-2 minutes until smooth.

5. Season with salt and pepper to taste. Serve warm.

Rich Turkey and Sweet Potato Blend

Prep Time: 15 mins | Cook Time: 40 mins | Serves: 4

Per Serving: Calories: 260 | Fat: 9g | Carbs: 35g | Fiber: 6g | Protein: 18g

Ingredients

- 1 lb ground turkey
- 2 medium sweet potatoes, peeled and chopped
- 1 small onion, chopped
- 1 cup low-sodium turkey or chicken broth
- 1 tbsp olive oil
- 1/4 tsp thyme
- Salt and pepper to taste

Procedure

1. Cook the sweet potatoes: Bring a pot of water to a boil. Add the chopped sweet potatoes and cook for 15-20 minutes until tender. Drain the water.

2. Cook the turkey: In a skillet, heat olive oil and cook the ground turkey with the chopped onion until the turkey is fully browned and cooked through (about 10 minutes).

3. Blend the ingredients: In a blender, combine the cooked sweet potatoes, turkey mixture, broth, and thyme. Blend until smooth.

4. Season with salt and pepper. Serve warm.

Dysphagia cookbook for beginners

Savory Beef and Mushroom Purée

Prep Time: 15 mins | Cook Time: 40 mins | Serves: 4

Per Serving: Calories: 290 | Fat: 12g | Carbs: 20g | Fiber: 4g | Protein: 25g

Ingredients

- 1 lb beef stew meat, cut into small cubes
- 1 cup mushrooms, sliced
- 1 small onion, chopped
- 1 garlic clove, minced
- 2 cups low-sodium beef broth
- 1 tbsp olive oil
- Salt and pepper to taste

Procedure

1. Cook the beef: In a large pot, heat the olive oil over medium heat. Add the beef and brown on all sides (about 5 minutes).

2. Add mushrooms and onions: Add the chopped mushrooms, onions, and garlic to the pot. Sauté for 5 minutes until softened.

3. Simmer the stew: Add the beef broth, reduce heat to low, and simmer for 30 minutes, until the beef is tender and fully cooked.

4. Blend the mixture: Transfer the entire stew to a blender and blend for 1-2 minutes until smooth.

5. Add salt and pepper to taste and serve warm.

Puréed Chicken Curry with Puréed Rice

Prep Time: 15 mins | Cook Time: 30 mins | Serves: 4

Per Serving: Calories: 350 | Fat: 15g | Carbs: 40g | Fiber: 5g | Protein: 20g

Ingredients

- 1 lb boneless, skinless chicken breast
- 1 cup cooked white rice (overcooked for softness)
- 1 small onion, chopped
- 1 garlic clove, minced
- 1 tbsp curry powder
- 1/2 tsp turmeric (optional)
- 1/2 cup coconut milk
- 1 cup low-sodium chicken broth
- 1 tbsp olive oil
- Salt and pepper to taste

Procedure

1. Cook the chicken: In a pot, bring water to a boil and add the chicken breast. Simmer for 15 minutes until fully cooked. Remove and set aside.

2. Prepare the curry sauce: In a skillet, heat olive oil and sauté the onions and garlic for 5 minutes. Add curry powder and turmeric, stirring to coat the onions.

3. Simmer the curry: Add coconut milk and chicken broth to the skillet and simmer for 10 minutes, allowing the flavors to meld.

4. Blend the chicken and curry: Transfer the cooked chicken and curry sauce to a blender. Blend until smooth.

5. Purée the rice: In the same blender, blend the overcooked rice with a little broth until smooth.

6. Serve the puréed chicken curry alongside the puréed rice.

Snacks and Light Meals

Puréed Cottage Cheese with Pureed Peaches

Prep Time: 5 mins | Cook Time: 0 mins | Serves: 2

Per Serving: Calories: 180 | Fat: 5g | Carbs: 20g | Fiber: 1g | Protein: 10g

Ingredients

- 1/2 cup low-fat cottage cheese
- 1/2 cup canned peaches in juice (drained)
- 1 tbsp honey (optional)

Procedure

1. Blend the cottage cheese: Place the cottage cheese in a blender and blend for 1-2 minutes until smooth and creamy.

2. Puree the peaches: In a separate blender or after cleaning the first, blend the canned peaches until smooth.

3. Combine: In a small bowl, layer the pureed cottage cheese with the pureed peaches.

4. Drizzle with honey for added sweetness (optional). Serve immediately.

Tropical Fruit Purée with Coconut

Prep Time: 10 mins | Cook Time: 0 mins | Serves: 2

Per Serving: Calories: 140 | Fat: 5g | Carbs: 25g | Fiber: 3g | Protein: 1g

Ingredients

- 1/2 cup fresh or canned pineapple, drained
- 1/2 cup mango, peeled and chopped
- 1 tbsp shredded coconut
- 1/4 cup coconut milk

Procedure

1. Blend the fruits: In a blender, combine the pineapple, mango, and coconut milk. Blend for 1-2 minutes until smooth.

2. Add coconut: Stir in the shredded coconut.

3. Pour into small bowls and enjoy chilled for a refreshing snack.

Peach Melba Pudding

Prep Time: 10 mins | Cook Time: 0 mins | Serves: 2

Per Serving: Calories: 200 | Fat: 7g | Carbs: 35g | Fiber: 3g | Protein: 3g

Ingredients

- 1 cup canned peaches in juice (drained)
- 1/4 cup raspberries (fresh or thawed from frozen)
- 1/4 cup Greek yogurt
- 1 tbsp honey (optional)

Procedure

1. Blend the peaches: In a blender, blend the peaches until smooth.
2. Blend the raspberries: Blend the raspberries separately until smooth.
3. Combine: In a small bowl, swirl together the peach puree, raspberry puree, and Greek yogurt.
4. Sweeten with honey if desired. Serve chilled.

Cinnamon Roll Apple Purée

Prep Time: 5 mins | Cook Time: 10 mins | Serves: 2

Per Serving: Calories: 160 | Fat: 3g | Carbs: 35g | Fiber: 4g | Protein: 1g

Ingredients

- 2 large apples, peeled and chopped
- 1 tsp cinnamon
- 1 tbsp honey
- 1/2 tsp vanilla extract

Procedure

1. Cook the apples: In a small saucepan, add the chopped apples with 1/4 cup of water. Cook over medium heat for about 10 minutes, until the apples are soft.
2. Blend the apples: Transfer the cooked apples to a blender. Add the cinnamon, honey, and vanilla extract. Blend until smooth.
3. Serve warm or chilled, depending on your preference.

Dysphagia cookbook for beginners

Puréed Avocado with Lime

Prep Time: 5 mins | Cook Time: 0 mins |
Serves: 2

Per Serving: Calories: 220 | Fat: 18g |
Carbs: 12g | Fiber: 6g | Protein: 2g

Ingredients

- 1 ripe avocado
- 1 tbsp lime juice
- 1 tbsp olive oil
- Salt to taste

Procedure

1. Prepare the avocado: Slice the avocado in half, remove the pit, and scoop the flesh into a blender.

2. Blend: Add the lime juice, olive oil, and a pinch of salt. Blend for 1-2 minutes until smooth and creamy.

3. Serve immediately as a snack or light meal.

Puréed Fruit Compote

Prep Time: 10 mins | Cook Time: 15 mins
| Serves: 4

Per Serving: Calories: 140 | Fat: 0g | Carbs: 35g | Fiber: 4g | Protein: 1g

Ingredients

- 2 apples, peeled and chopped
- 2 pears, peeled and chopped
- 1/2 cup water
- 1/4 tsp cinnamon
- 1 tbsp honey (optional)

Procedure

1. Cook the fruits: In a medium saucepan, combine the apples, pears, and water. Bring to a boil, reduce heat, and simmer for 10-15 minutes, until the fruit is soft.

2. Blend the fruits: Transfer the cooked fruit to a blender. Add the cinnamon and honey, then blend until smooth.

3. Serve warm or chilled, depending on your preference.

Blended Rice Pudding

Prep Time: 5 mins | Cook Time: 25 mins | Serves: 4

Per Serving: Calories: 250 | Fat: 6g | Carbs: 45g | Fiber: 1g | Protein: 7g

Ingredients

- 1/2 cup white rice
- 2 cups milk
- 1/4 cup sugar
- 1 tsp vanilla extract
- 1/2 tsp cinnamon

Procedure

1. Cook the rice: In a medium pot, combine the rice and milk. Bring to a simmer and cook for about 20-25 minutes, until the rice is soft and the mixture has thickened.

2. Sweeten the pudding: Stir in the sugar, vanilla extract, and cinnamon. Mix well and cook for another 2 minutes.

3. Blend: Transfer the cooked rice pudding to a blender and blend until smooth.

4. Serve warm or chilled.

Puréed Mango with Coconut Milk

Prep Time: 5 mins | Cook Time: 0 mins | Serves: 2

Per Serving: Calories: 160 | Fat: 7g | Carbs: 25g | Fiber: 3g | Protein: 2g

Ingredients

- 1 ripe mango, peeled and chopped
- 1/2 cup coconut milk
- 1 tbsp honey (optional)

Procedure

1. Blend the mango: In a blender, combine the mango and coconut milk. Blend for 1-2 minutes until smooth.

2. Sweeten: Add honey for extra sweetness if desired and blend briefly to combine.

3. Pour into small bowls and enjoy chilled.

Puréed Rice Pudding

Prep Time: 5 mins | Cook Time: 25 mins | Serves: 4

Per Serving: Calories: 230 | Fat: 6g | Carbs: 40g | Fiber: 1g | Protein: 6g

Ingredients

- 1/2 cup white rice
- 2 cups milk
- 1/4 cup sugar
- 1 tsp vanilla extract
- 1/2 tsp cinnamon

Procedure

1. Cook the rice: In a pot, combine the rice and milk. Bring to a simmer over medium heat and cook for about 20-25 minutes, stirring occasionally, until the rice is soft and the pudding thickens.
2. Sweeten: Stir in the sugar, vanilla, and cinnamon, mixing well.
3. Blend the pudding: Transfer the rice pudding to a blender and blend until smooth and creamy.
4. Serve warm or chilled.

Creamy Custard with Puréed Fruit

Prep Time: 5 mins | Cook Time: 10 mins | Serves: 4

Per Serving: Calories: 200 | Fat: 8g | Carbs: 30g | Fiber: 1g | Protein: 5g

Ingredients

- 2 cups milk
- 2 tbsp cornstarch
- 1/4 cup sugar
- 1 tsp vanilla extract
- 1/2 cup pureed fruit (such as strawberries, peaches, or raspberries)

Procedure

1. Make the custard: In a small saucepan, whisk together the milk, cornstarch, and sugar. Cook over medium heat, stirring constantly, until the mixture thickens (about 5-10 minutes). Remove from heat and stir in the vanilla.
2. Cool the custard: Let the custard cool slightly before blending.
3. Combine: In a blender, blend the cooled custard and pureed fruit until smooth.
4. Serve warm or chilled, depending on your preference.

Meal plan

Day 1

- Breakfast: Creamy Banana and Peanut Butter Oatmeal
- Lunch: Puréed Chicken and Vegetable Soup
- Dinner: Puréed Spinach and Ricotta Lasagna
- Snack: Tropical Fruit Purée with Coconut

Day 2

- Breakfast: Lemon Ricotta Pancake Purée
- Lunch: Creamy Mashed Potatoes with Soft Meatloaf Purée
- Dinner: Puréed Beef Stew with Root Vegetables
- Snack: Puréed Mango with Coconut Milk

Day 3

- Breakfast: Savory Tomato Basil Omelette Purée
- Lunch: Puréed Avocado Toast
- Dinner: Puréed Chicken Alfredo with Puréed Broccoli
- Snack: Blended Rice Pudding

Day 4

- Breakfast: Creamy Oatmeal
- Lunch: Puréed Vegetable Medley with Soft-Cooked Lentils
- Dinner: Carrot and Ginger Soup with Puréed Chicken
- Snack: Puréed Cottage Cheese with Puréed Peaches

Day 5

- Breakfast: Peaches and Cream Purée
- Lunch: Puréed Macaroni and Cheese
- Dinner: Puréed Meatloaf with Puréed Carrots
- Snack: Cinnamon Roll Apple Purée

Day 6

- Breakfast: Puréed Fruit Smoothie
- Lunch: Puréed Chicken Curry with Puréed Rice
- Dinner: Spaghetti Bolognese Puréed
- Snack: Peach Melba Pudding

Day 7

- Breakfast: Puréed Mango Coconut Rice Pudding
- Lunch: Rich Turkey and Sweet Potato Blend
- Dinner: Savory Beef and Mushroom Purée
- Snack: Puréed Fruit Compote

Chapter 4

Level 2: Mechanically Altered/Soft Foods (Some Chewing Required)

Mashed Berry Parfait with Soft Oats Layers

Prep Time: 10 mins | Cook Time: 5 mins | Serves: 2
Per Serving: Calories: 180 | Fat: 4g | Carbs: 30g | Fiber: 5g | Protein: 6g

Ingredients

- 1/2 cup rolled oats
- 1/2 cup milk
- 1/2 cup mixed berries (soft, ripe, or thawed frozen berries)
- 1 tbsp honey (optional)
- 1/4 cup Greek yogurt

Procedure

1. Cook the oats: In a small saucepan, cook the oats in milk over medium heat for 3-5 minutes until soft.

2. Mash the berries: In a bowl, mash the berries with a fork or blender until they are smooth but retain some texture.

3. Layer the parfait: In small serving glasses, layer the cooked oats, mashed berries, and Greek yogurt.

4. Sweeten with honey if desired and serve immediately.

Minced Egg and Cheese Breakfast Burrito

(Using Soft Tortillas)

Prep Time: 10 mins | Cook Time: 10 mins | Serves: 2

Per Serving: Calories: 300 | Fat: 16g | Carbs: 25g | Fiber: 3g | Protein: 16g

Ingredients

- 4 eggs, scrambled

- 1/4 cup shredded cheddar cheese

- 2 soft flour tortillas

- 1 tbsp butter

- 1/4 cup minced tomatoes (optional)

Procedure

1. Cook the eggs: In a non-stick skillet, melt the butter and scramble the eggs until fully cooked but soft.

2. Assemble the burrito: On each soft tortilla, place half the scrambled eggs, shredded cheese, and minced tomatoes.

3. Fold the tortilla into a burrito shape. Cut into small, bite-sized pieces for easy chewing. Serve warm.

Dysphagia cookbook for beginners

Turkey Sausage with Soft Polenta

Prep Time: 15 mins | Cook Time: 20 mins | Serves: 2
Per Serving: Calories: 290 | Fat: 15g | Carbs: 25g | Fiber: 3g | Protein: 18g

Ingredients

- 2 turkey sausages (minced)
- 1/2 cup polenta (cornmeal)
- 1 1/2 cups water or low-sodium broth
- 1 tbsp butter
- Salt and pepper to taste

Procedure

1. Cook the polenta: In a saucepan, bring the water or broth to a boil. Slowly whisk in the polenta and cook for 10-15 minutes, stirring often, until soft and creamy. Add the butter, salt, and pepper.

2. Cook and mince the sausage: While the polenta is cooking, grill or cook the turkey sausages in a skillet. Once cooked, mince the sausage into small pieces.

3. Serve the minced turkey sausage over the soft polenta. Ensure the sausage pieces are small and soft enough for easy chewing.

Minced Soft Baked Apples with Cinnamon

Prep Time: 10 mins | Cook Time: 20 mins | Serves: 2

Per Serving: Calories: 150 | Fat: 3g | Carbs: 35g | Fiber: 5g | Protein: 1g

Ingredients

- 2 large apples, peeled, cored, and chopped
- 1 tbsp honey
- 1/2 tsp cinnamon
- 1 tbsp butter

Procedure

1. Bake the apples: Preheat the oven to 350°F (175°C). Place the chopped apples in a baking dish, sprinkle with cinnamon, and dot with butter. Cover with foil and bake for 20 minutes, until the apples are soft.

2. Mash or mince: Once the apples are baked, mash or mince them into small, soft pieces.

3. Drizzle with honey if desired and serve warm.

Minced Huevos Rancheros with Avocado

Prep Time: 15 mins | Cook Time: 10 mins | Serves: 2
Per Serving: Calories: 250 | Fat: 18g | Carbs: 15g | Fiber: 5g | Protein: 10g

Ingredients

- 2 eggs, scrambled
- 1/2 avocado, mashed
- 1 soft corn tortilla
- 1/4 cup minced tomatoes
- 1 tbsp minced onions
- 1 tbsp olive oil
- Salt and pepper to taste

Procedure

1. Prepare the scrambled eggs: In a skillet, heat olive oil and scramble the eggs until soft.

2. Soften the tortilla: Warm the soft tortilla in the microwave for 10-15 seconds or until pliable.

3. Assemble: On the tortilla, spread the mashed avocado, followed by the scrambled eggs, minced tomatoes, and onions.

4. Mince the entire dish into small, manageable pieces before serving.

Minced Tofu Scramble with Soft Veggies

Prep Time: 10 mins | Cook Time: 15 mins | Serves: 2

Per Serving: Calories: 220 | Fat: 10g | Carbs: 12g | Fiber: 3g | Protein: 20g

Ingredients

- 1/2 block firm tofu, crumbled
- 1/4 cup minced spinach (cooked and soft)
- 1/4 cup minced soft vegetables (zucchini or bell peppers)
- 1 tsp turmeric (optional for color)
- 1 tbsp olive oil
- Salt and pepper to taste

Procedure

1. Cook the tofu: In a skillet, heat the olive oil over medium heat. Add the crumbled tofu and cook for 5 minutes, stirring occasionally.

2. Add the vegetables: Stir in the minced spinach and soft vegetables. Cook for another 5 minutes until the vegetables are soft and the tofu is fully cooked.

3. Season with salt, pepper, and turmeric (optional). Mince the tofu scramble if needed for easier chewing. Serve warm.

Mashed Bean and Vegetable Casserole

Prep Time: 15 mins | Cook Time: 30 mins | Serves: 4

Per Serving: Calories: 250 | Fat: 8g | Carbs: 35g | Fiber: 8g | Protein: 10g

Ingredients

- 1 cup canned beans (kidney, black, or pinto), rinsed and mashed
- 1 cup soft-cooked vegetables (carrots, zucchini, or spinach), finely minced
- 1/2 cup vegetable broth
- 1/2 cup shredded cheese (optional)
- 1/4 cup breadcrumbs (optional)
- 1 tbsp olive oil
- Salt and pepper to taste

Procedure

1. Prepare the vegetables: In a skillet, heat the olive oil over medium heat. Add the minced vegetables and sauté for 5-7 minutes, until soft.

2. Mash the beans: In a bowl, mash the beans with a fork or potato masher until smooth but slightly textured.

3. Combine and bake: Mix the mashed beans, cooked vegetables, and vegetable broth in a baking dish. Sprinkle shredded cheese and breadcrumbs on top if using.

4. Bake: Preheat the oven to 350°F (175°C). Bake for 20 minutes, until the top is golden and the mixture is heated through.

5. Let cool slightly before serving. The casserole should be soft with mashed textures.

Minced Sweet Potato Hash with Soft Poached Eggs

Prep Time: 15 mins | Cook Time: 20 mins | Serves: 2
Per Serving: Calories: 280 | Fat: 12g | Carbs: 35g | Fiber: 5g | Protein: 10g

Ingredients

- 2 medium sweet potatoes, peeled and chopped
- 1/4 cup minced onion
- 1 tbsp olive oil
- 2 eggs
- Salt and pepper to taste

Procedure

1. Cook the sweet potatoes: In a skillet, heat the olive oil over medium heat. Add the chopped sweet potatoes and onion, and cook for 15-20 minutes, stirring occasionally, until the sweet potatoes are soft.

2. Mash or mince: Lightly mash the sweet potatoes with a fork or mince them into small, soft pieces for easier chewing.

3. Poach the eggs: In a small pot, bring water to a simmer. Crack the eggs into the water and poach for 3-4 minutes, until the whites are set but the yolks remain soft.

4. Place the mashed sweet potato hash on a plate and top with the poached eggs. Season with salt and pepper.

Softened Rice Pudding with Softened Raisins

Prep Time: 10 mins | Cook Time: 25 mins | Serves: 4

Per Serving: Calories: 220 | Fat: 5g | Carbs: 40g | Fiber: 2g | Protein: 6g

Ingredients

- 1/2 cup white rice
- 2 cups milk
- 1/4 cup sugar
- 1 tsp vanilla extract
- 1/4 cup raisins (softened by soaking in warm water for 10 minutes)
- 1/2 tsp cinnamon

Procedure

1. Cook the rice: In a medium saucepan, combine the rice and milk. Cook over medium heat for about 20 minutes, stirring occasionally, until the rice is soft and the mixture has thickened.

2. Add the raisins: Drain the softened raisins and stir them into the rice pudding.

3. Sweeten the pudding: Add the sugar, vanilla, and cinnamon, mixing well. Cook for an additional 2-3 minutes.

4. Serve warm or chilled. The pudding should be soft with no hard or chewy textures.

Minced Creamy Ricotta with Softened Pears

Prep Time: 5 mins | Cook Time: 10 mins | Serves: 2

Per Serving: Calories: 180 | Fat: 6g | Carbs: 25g | Fiber: 3g | Protein: 6g

Ingredients

- 1/2 cup ricotta cheese
- 2 ripe pears, peeled and chopped
- 1 tbsp honey (optional)
- 1/4 tsp cinnamon

Procedure

1. Soften the pears: In a small saucepan, cook the chopped pears with 1/4 cup water over medium heat for about 10 minutes, until the pears are soft and easily mashed.

2. Mash the pears: Mash the softened pears with a fork or mince them into small, soft pieces.

3. Combine with ricotta: In a bowl, mix the mashed pears with the ricotta cheese.

4. Drizzle with honey and sprinkle with cinnamon if desired. Serve immediately as a light, soft breakfast.

Easy Lunch ideas

Soft Lentil and Vegetable Soup

Prep Time: 10 mins | Cook Time: 30 mins | Serves: 4
Per Serving: Calories: 220 | Fat: 5g | Carbs: 35g | Fiber: 8g | Protein: 10g

Ingredients

- 1 cup red or green lentils, rinsed
- 1 carrot, finely chopped
- 1 small onion, minced
- 1 celery stalk, minced
- 4 cups low-sodium vegetable broth
- 1 tbsp olive oil
- Salt and pepper to taste

Procedure

1. Sauté the vegetables: In a large pot, heat the olive oil over medium heat. Add the minced onion, carrot, and celery, and cook for 5 minutes until softened.

2. Cook the lentils: Add the lentils and broth to the pot. Bring to a boil, then reduce the heat and simmer for 20-25 minutes, until the lentils are soft.

3. Mash or blend: For a smoother texture, mash some of the lentils or use a hand blender to blend part of the soup while leaving some texture intact.

4. Season with salt and pepper to taste. Serve warm.

Minced Shepherd's Pie

(Soft Mashed Topping)

Prep Time: 20 mins | Cook Time: 40 mins | Serves: 4

Per Serving: Calories: 350 | Fat: 15g | Carbs: 40g | Fiber: 5g | Protein: 20g

Ingredients

- 1 lb ground beef or turkey, minced
- 2 medium potatoes, peeled and mashed
- 1/2 cup mixed soft vegetables (carrots, peas, and corn), minced
- 1/4 cup low-sodium beef broth
- 1 tbsp butter
- Salt and pepper to taste

Procedure

1. Cook the meat: In a skillet, brown the minced ground beef or turkey over medium heat. Drain any excess fat.

2. Cook the vegetables: Mince the vegetables finely and add them to the skillet with the meat. Add the broth and simmer for 5 minutes until the vegetables are soft.

3. Mash the potatoes: Boil the peeled potatoes in water until tender, then mash with butter and salt until smooth.

4. Assemble: In a baking dish, spread the meat and vegetable mixture evenly. Top with the mashed potatoes.

5. Bake: Preheat the oven to 350°F (175°C) and bake for 20 minutes, until the top is golden.

6. Let cool slightly and serve. Mince or mash further if needed for easier chewing.

Minced Soft Beef Tacos

(Using Soft Tortillas)

Prep Time: 10 mins | Cook Time: 10 mins | Serves: 4

Per Serving: Calories: 320 | Fat: 16g | Carbs: 30g | Fiber: 3g | Protein: 20g

Ingredients

- 1 lb ground beef, cooked and minced

- 1/4 cup minced tomatoes

- 1/4 cup shredded cheese

- 4 soft flour tortillas

- 1 tbsp olive oil

- 1 tbsp taco seasoning (optional)

Procedure

1. Cook the beef: In a skillet, heat the olive oil over medium heat. Add the ground beef and taco seasoning (if using) and cook until browned. Mince the beef into small pieces.

2. Warm the tortillas: Warm the soft tortillas in the microwave for 10-15 seconds to soften them.

3. Assemble the tacos: Spoon the minced beef onto each tortilla. Top with minced tomatoes and shredded cheese.

4. Fold the tortillas and serve. Cut into smaller pieces if necessary for easier chewing.

Minced Vegetable Stir-fry with Soft Tofu

Prep Time: 15 mins | Cook Time: 10 mins | Serves: 4

Per Serving: Calories: 200 | Fat: 10g | Carbs: 20g | Fiber: 5g | Protein: 12g

Ingredients

- 1/2 block soft tofu, cut into small cubes
- 1 cup soft vegetables (carrots, zucchini, bell peppers), minced
- 1 tbsp soy sauce (low sodium)
- 1 tbsp olive oil
- 1/4 tsp ginger (optional)

Procedure

1. Sauté the vegetables: In a skillet, heat the olive oil over medium heat. Add the minced vegetables and ginger, and sauté for 5-7 minutes until the vegetables are soft.

2. Add tofu and soy sauce: Add the soft tofu cubes to the skillet, and drizzle with soy sauce. Cook for an additional 2-3 minutes, until heated through.

3. Serve immediately. Ensure the tofu and vegetables are minced small enough for easy chewing.

Soft Barley and Mushroom Soup

Prep Time: 10 mins | Cook Time: 45 mins | Serves: 4
Per Serving: Calories: 230 | Fat: 6g | Carbs: 35g | Fiber: 5g | Protein: 8g

Ingredients

- 1/2 cup pearl barley
- 1 cup mushrooms, finely chopped
- 1 small onion, minced
- 4 cups low-sodium vegetable broth
- 1 tbsp olive oil
- Salt and pepper to taste

Procedure

1. Cook the barley: In a large pot, combine the barley and vegetable broth. Bring to a boil, then reduce heat and simmer for 30-35 minutes, until the barley is soft.

2. Sauté the mushrooms: In a separate skillet, heat olive oil and sauté the minced mushrooms and onions for 5 minutes until soft.

3. Combine: Add the mushroom mixture to the pot with the barley and simmer for an additional 10 minutes.

4. Serve warm. You can mash or blend part of the soup for a smoother consistency.

Minced Chicken Alfredo with Softened Pasta

Prep Time: 15 mins | Cook Time: 25 mins | Serves: 4

Per Serving: Calories: 450 | Fat: 20g | Carbs: 40g | Fiber: 3g | Protein: 25g

Ingredients

- 1 lb boneless, skinless chicken breast, minced
- 6 oz soft pasta (such as fettuccine or penne), cooked very soft
- 1/2 cup heavy cream
- 1/2 cup grated Parmesan cheese
- 1 tbsp butter
- Salt and pepper to taste

Procedure

1. Cook the pasta: Cook the pasta until very soft (beyond al dente), then drain and set aside.

2. Cook and mince the chicken: In a skillet, cook the chicken breast over medium heat until fully cooked. Mince the chicken into small pieces.

3. Prepare the Alfredo sauce: In a separate saucepan, melt the butter over low heat. Stir in the heavy cream and Parmesan cheese, and cook until the sauce thickens.

4. Add the cooked pasta and minced chicken to the sauce, stirring gently to combine. Serve warm.

Minced Soft Meat Lasagna

(Soft Layers, Minced Filling)

Prep Time: 20 mins | Cook Time: 45 mins | Serves: 4

Per Serving: Calories: 450 | Fat: 20g | Carbs: 40g | Fiber: 5g | Protein: 25g

Ingredients

- 6 soft lasagna noodles, cooked very soft
- 1 lb ground beef or turkey, minced
- 1/2 cup marinara sauce (smooth, no chunks)
- 1/2 cup ricotta cheese
- 1/4 cup shredded mozzarella cheese
- 1 tbsp olive oil
- Salt and pepper to taste

Procedure

1. Cook the lasagna noodles: Boil the lasagna noodles until very soft. Drain and set aside.

2. Cook and mince the meat: In a skillet, heat olive oil over medium heat. Add the ground meat and cook until browned. Mince the cooked meat into very small pieces using a food processor or by hand.

3. Assemble the lasagna: In a greased baking dish, layer the soft lasagna noodles, minced meat, ricotta cheese, and marinara sauce. Repeat the layers.

4. Top with mozzarella: Sprinkle shredded mozzarella on top.

5. Bake: Preheat the oven to 350°F (175°C) and bake for 20-25 minutes, until the cheese is melted and bubbly.

6. Let cool slightly before serving. Cut into small, manageable pieces if necessary.

Soft-Cooked Carrot and Swede Mash

Prep Time: 10 mins | Cook Time: 20 mins | Serves: 4

Per Serving: Calories: 120 | Fat: 4g | Carbs: 20g | Fiber: 5g | Protein: 2g

Ingredients

- 2 large carrots, peeled and chopped
- 1 large swede (rutabaga), peeled and chopped
- 1 tbsp butter
- Salt and pepper to taste

Procedure

1. Cook the vegetables: Bring a large pot of water to a boil. Add the chopped carrots and swede and cook for 15-20 minutes, until soft and tender.

2. Mash the vegetables: Drain the water and mash the cooked carrots and swede together with a fork or potato masher until smooth.

3. Add butter: Stir in the butter, salt, and pepper.

4. Serve warm as a side dish. Mince further if needed for easier chewing.

Minced Soft Salmon Cakes with Soft Vegetables

Prep Time: 15 mins | Cook Time: 10 mins | Serves: 4
Per Serving: Calories: 300 | Fat: 15g | Carbs: 20g | Fiber: 3g | Protein: 25g

Ingredients

- 1 lb cooked salmon, minced
- 1/2 cup breadcrumbs (softened)
- 1 egg, beaten
- 1/4 cup mayonnaise
- 1 tbsp lemon juice
- 1 cup soft vegetables (e.g., carrots, peas), cooked and minced
- 1 tbsp olive oil
- Salt and pepper to taste

Procedure

1. Prepare the salmon mixture: In a bowl, combine the minced salmon, breadcrumbs, egg, mayonnaise, and lemon juice. Mix well.

2. Form the cakes: Shape the mixture into small patties.

3. Cook the salmon cakes: Heat olive oil in a skillet over medium heat. Cook the salmon cakes for 3-4 minutes on each side until golden brown and heated through.

4. Cook the vegetables: While the salmon cakes are cooking, steam or boil the soft vegetables until tender. Mince them into small pieces.

5. Serve the salmon cakes with the minced soft vegetables on the side.

Soft Blended Avocado Toast

Prep Time: 5 mins | Cook Time: 0 mins | Serves: 2

Per Serving: Calories: 220 | Fat: 18g | Carbs: 12g | Fiber: 6g | Protein: 4g

Ingredients

- 1 ripe avocado
- 2 slices soft sandwich bread
- 1 tbsp olive oil
- 1 tbsp lemon juice
- Salt to taste

Procedure

1. Prepare the avocado: Slice the avocado in half, remove the pit, and scoop the flesh into a blender.

2. Blend: Add the olive oil, lemon juice, and salt. Blend until smooth.

3. Toast the bread: Toast the soft bread slices lightly, or skip toasting if needed for softer texture.

4. Spread the avocado: Spread the blended avocado on the bread slices. Cut into small, manageable pieces if needed.

5. Serve immediately.

Dinner ideas

Minced Soft Beef Stroganoff with Soft Noodles

Prep Time: 15 mins | Cook Time: 30 mins | Serves: 4

Per Serving: Calories: 400 | Fat: 20g | Carbs: 35g | Fiber: 4g | Protein: 25g

Ingredients

- 1 lb ground beef, minced
- 1 small onion, minced
- 1/2 cup mushrooms, minced
- 1 cup sour cream
- 1/4 cup beef broth
- 6 oz soft egg noodles, cooked very soft
- 1 tbsp olive oil
- Salt and pepper to taste

Procedure

1. Cook the beef: In a large skillet, heat olive oil over medium heat. Add the minced beef, onion, and mushrooms. Cook for 10 minutes until browned and soft.

2. Prepare the sauce: Add the beef broth and sour cream to the skillet, stirring to combine. Simmer for an additional 5-7 minutes until the sauce thickens slightly.

3. Cook the noodles: Cook the egg noodles in boiling water until very soft, then drain.

4. Add the soft noodles to the skillet and toss gently to coat in the stroganoff sauce. Serve warm.

Mashed Chickpea and Roasted Vegetable Bowl

Prep Time: 15 mins | Cook Time: 30 mins | Serves: 4

Per Serving: Calories: 320 | Fat: 10g | Carbs: 45g | Fiber: 10g | Protein: 12g

Ingredients

- 1 can chickpeas, rinsed and mashed
- 1 zucchini, chopped and roasted
- 1 carrot, chopped and roasted
- 1/4 cup olive oil
- 1 tbsp tahini (optional)
- Salt and pepper to taste

Procedure

1. Roast the vegetables: Preheat the oven to 400°F (200°C). Toss the chopped zucchini and carrot with olive oil, salt, and pepper. Roast for 20-25 minutes, until soft.

2. Mash the chickpeas: In a bowl, mash the chickpeas with a fork or potato masher until smooth but slightly textured. Add tahini if desired for creaminess.

3. Layer the mashed chickpeas in a bowl and top with the roasted vegetables. Drizzle with extra olive oil if needed and serve.

Minced Chicken with Olive Tapenade

Prep Time: 15 mins | Cook Time: 20 mins | Serves: 4

Per Serving: Calories: 280 | Fat: 15g | Carbs: 5g | Fiber: 2g | Protein: 25g

Ingredients

- 1 lb chicken breast, minced
- 1/2 cup olive tapenade (store-bought or homemade)
- 1 tbsp olive oil
- 1/4 tsp garlic powder
- Salt and pepper to taste

Procedure

1. Cook the chicken: In a skillet, heat olive oil over medium heat. Add the minced chicken and cook for 10-12 minutes until fully cooked. Season with garlic powder, salt, and pepper.

2. Add the tapenade: Stir in the olive tapenade and cook for an additional 2-3 minutes to warm through.

3. Serve warm as a topping for soft bread or alongside soft-cooked vegetables.

Minced Beef and Eggplant Purée

Prep Time: 15 mins | Cook Time: 30 mins | Serves: 4

Per Serving: Calories: 350 | Fat: 18g | Carbs: 25g | Fiber: 7g | Protein: 20g

Ingredients

- 1 lb ground beef, minced
- 1 large eggplant, peeled and chopped
- 1 small onion, minced
- 1/2 cup low-sodium beef broth
- 1 tbsp olive oil
- Salt and pepper to taste

Procedure

1. Cook the eggplant: In a large pot, bring water to a boil. Add the chopped eggplant and cook for 15 minutes, until soft. Drain and set aside.

2. Cook the beef: In a skillet, heat olive oil over medium heat. Add the minced beef and onion, cooking until browned and fully cooked (about 10 minutes).

3. Blend the eggplant: Blend the cooked eggplant with the beef broth until smooth.

4. Combine: Stir the pureed eggplant into the minced beef mixture, season with salt and pepper, and cook for another 5 minutes.

5. Serve warm.

Seafood Chowder Soup

Prep Time: 20 mins | Cook Time: 30 mins | Serves: 4

Per Serving: Calories: 300 | Fat: 12g | Carbs: 30g | Fiber: 3g | Protein: 20g

Ingredients

- 1/2 lb white fish (cod or haddock), minced
- 1/2 lb shrimp, minced
- 1 large potato, peeled and chopped
- 1 small onion, minced
- 2 cups low-sodium vegetable or seafood broth
- 1 cup milk
- 1 tbsp butter
- 1/4 tsp thyme
- Salt and pepper to taste

Procedure

1. Cook the vegetables: In a large pot, melt the butter over medium heat. Add the minced onion and chopped potato, cooking for 5 minutes.

2. Add the broth: Pour in the vegetable or seafood broth and bring to a simmer. Cook for 15 minutes until the potatoes are soft.

3. Add seafood: Stir in the minced fish and shrimp, cooking for another 10 minutes until the seafood is fully cooked.

4. Finish with milk: Stir in the milk and thyme, allowing the soup to heat through for 5 minutes.

5. Season with salt and pepper, and serve warm.

Minced Meatloaf with Soft Cooked Carrots

Prep Time: 20 mins | Cook Time: 40 mins | Serves: 4
Per Serving: Calories: 320 | Fat: 15g | Carbs: 25g | Fiber: 5g | Protein: 20g

Ingredients

- 1 lb ground beef or turkey, minced
- 1/4 cup breadcrumbs (softened)
- 1 egg, beaten
- 1/4 cup ketchup
- 1 tbsp Worcestershire sauce (optional)
- 4 large carrots, peeled and chopped
- 1 tbsp butter
- Salt and pepper to taste

Procedure

1. Prepare the meatloaf mixture: In a mixing bowl, combine the minced ground meat, breadcrumbs, beaten egg, ketchup, Worcestershire sauce (if using), salt, and pepper. Mix well.

2. Form and bake the meatloaf: Shape the meat mixture into a loaf and place it in a greased loaf pan. Bake at 350°F (175°C) for 35-40 minutes, until fully cooked.

3. Cook the carrots: While the meatloaf is baking, bring a pot of water to a boil. Add the chopped carrots and cook for 15-20 minutes until soft. Drain, then mash the carrots with butter.

4. Mince the meatloaf: Once the meatloaf is cooked, allow it to cool slightly. Mince or finely chop the meatloaf for easier chewing.

5. Serve the minced meatloaf with the soft mashed carrots on the side.

Minced Turkey Shepherd's Pie

(Soft Mashed Potato Topping)

Prep Time: 20 mins | Cook Time: 35 mins | Serves: 4

Per Serving: Calories: 350 | Fat: 12g | Carbs: 40g | Fiber: 5g | Protein: 20g

Ingredients

- 1 lb ground turkey, minced
- 2 medium potatoes, peeled and chopped
- 1/2 cup soft vegetables (peas, carrots), finely minced
- 1/4 cup low-sodium turkey broth
- 1 tbsp butter
- Salt and pepper to taste

Procedure

1. Cook the ground turkey: In a skillet, cook the minced ground turkey until browned and fully cooked, about 10 minutes.

2. Cook the vegetables: Mince the soft vegetables (such as carrots and peas) finely and add to the cooked turkey. Add the broth and simmer for 5 minutes until the vegetables are soft.

3. Mash the potatoes: Boil the potatoes in water until tender, about 15 minutes. Drain and mash with butter and a little salt.

4. Assemble the Shepherd's Pie: In a greased baking dish, layer the turkey and vegetable mixture, and top with the soft mashed potatoes.

5. Bake: Preheat the oven to 350°F (175°C) and bake for 15-20 minutes until the top is golden.

6. Let cool slightly and serve in small, minced portions.

Minced Chicken and Dumplings
(Soft Dumplings)

Prep Time: 15 mins | Cook Time: 30 mins | Serves: 4

Per Serving: Calories: 320 | Fat: 12g | Carbs: 35g | Fiber: 4g | Protein: 20g

Ingredients

- 1 lb chicken breast, minced
- 1 small onion, minced
- 2 carrots, peeled and minced
- 1/2 cup low-sodium chicken broth
- 1 cup flour
- 1/2 cup milk
- 1 tbsp butter
- Salt and pepper to taste

Procedure

1. Prepare the chicken and vegetables: In a large pot, sauté the minced onion and carrots in butter until soft, about 5 minutes. Add the minced chicken and cook until browned.

2. Add broth and simmer: Pour in the chicken broth and simmer for 10 minutes, until the mixture is heated through.

3. Prepare the dumplings: In a bowl, mix the flour, milk, and a pinch of salt until a soft dough forms. Using a spoon, drop small spoonfuls of dough into the simmering broth.

4. Cook the dumplings: Cover the pot and cook the dumplings for 10-12 minutes, until they are soft and fully cooked.

5. Mince or mash the dumplings if necessary, and serve the dish warm.

Minced Soft Turkey with Stuffing and Gravy

Prep Time: 20 mins | Cook Time: 25 mins | Serves: 4

Per Serving: Calories: 350 | Fat: 14g | Carbs: 30g | Fiber: 3g | Protein: 25g

Ingredients

- 1 lb cooked turkey breast, minced
- 1/2 cup soft stuffing (prepared from mix or homemade)
- 1/2 cup low-sodium turkey gravy
- 1 tbsp olive oil
- 1/2 tsp dried sage (optional)

Procedure

1. Mince the turkey: Mince the cooked turkey breast into small, manageable pieces.

2. Prepare the stuffing: Prepare soft stuffing using a pre-made mix or homemade recipe, ensuring the texture is moist and easy to chew.

3. Combine and heat: In a skillet, heat the olive oil over medium heat. Add the minced turkey, stuffing, and gravy. Cook for 5-7 minutes until everything is warmed through.

4. Add a sprinkle of sage if desired and serve warm.

Minced Soft Pasta Carbonara with Soft Bacon

Prep Time: 15 mins | Cook Time: 15 mins | Serves: 4

Per Serving: Calories: 450 | Fat: 22g | Carbs: 45g | Fiber: 2g | Protein: 20g

Ingredients

- 6 oz soft pasta (such as fettuccine or penne), cooked very soft
- 1/4 cup grated Parmesan cheese
- 2 large eggs, beaten
- 4 slices soft-cooked bacon, minced
- 1/4 cup cream
- 1 tbsp butter
- Salt and pepper to taste

Procedure

1. Cook the pasta: Cook the pasta in boiling water until very soft, then drain and set aside.

2. Cook the bacon: Cook the bacon in a skillet over medium heat until soft but not crispy. Mince the bacon into small pieces.

3. Prepare the carbonara sauce: In a small saucepan, heat the butter and cream over low heat. Stir in the beaten eggs and Parmesan cheese, whisking constantly until the sauce thickens.

4. Combine the pasta and sauce: Add the soft pasta and minced bacon to the saucepan, stirring gently to coat everything in the sauce.

5. Season with salt and pepper and serve warm.

Tasty Snack

Honeyed Pear Purée

Prep Time: 5 mins | Cook Time: 10 mins | Serves: 2

Per Serving: Calories: 150 | Fat: 1g | Carbs: 38g | Fiber: 5g | Protein: 1g

Ingredients

- 2 ripe pears, peeled and chopped
- 1 tbsp honey
- 1/4 tsp cinnamon (optional)
- 1/4 cup water

Procedure

1. Cook the pears: In a small saucepan, combine the chopped pears, water, and honey. Cook over medium heat for about 10 minutes, or until the pears are soft and easily mashed.

2. Blend or mash: Transfer the cooked pears to a blender and blend until smooth. Alternatively, you can mash the pears with a fork for a chunkier texture.

3. Sprinkle with cinnamon if desired. Serve warm or chilled.

Soft Baked Apple Slices

Prep Time: 5 mins | Cook Time: 20 mins | Serves: 2

Per Serving: Calories: 140 | Fat: 3g | Carbs: 30g | Fiber: 4g | Protein: 1g

Ingredients

- 2 large apples, peeled and sliced
- 1 tbsp butter
- 1 tbsp honey
- 1/2 tsp cinnamon

Procedure

1. Prepare the apples: Preheat the oven to 350°F (175°C). In a baking dish, arrange the peeled and sliced apples.

2. Add flavor: Dot the apple slices with butter and drizzle with honey. Sprinkle the cinnamon on top.

3. Bake the apples: Cover the dish with foil and bake for 20 minutes, or until the apples are very soft.

4. Serve warm as a soft, flavorful dessert or snack.

Minced Soft Fruit Smoothie

(Using Soft Fruits Like Bananas or Peaches)

Prep Time: 5 mins | Cook Time: 0 mins | Serves: 2

Per Serving: Calories: 180 | Fat: 2g | Carbs: 40g | Fiber: 4g | Protein: 3g

Ingredients

- 1 ripe banana, peeled and chopped
- 1/2 cup ripe peaches, peeled and chopped (fresh or canned in juice)
- 1/2 cup plain yogurt or milk
- 1 tbsp honey (optional)
- 1/4 tsp vanilla extract (optional)

Procedure

1. Prepare the fruits: Peel and chop the banana and peaches.

2. Blend: Place the soft fruits in a blender along with yogurt (or milk), honey, and vanilla extract. Blend until smooth.

3. Pour into glasses and enjoy as a refreshing soft smoothie. Serve chilled.

Banana Foster Purée

Prep Time: 5 mins | Cook Time: 10 mins | Serves: 2
Per Serving: Calories: 220 | Fat: 8g | Carbs: 35g | Fiber: 3g | Protein: 2g

Ingredients

- 2 ripe bananas, sliced
- 1 tbsp butter
- 1 tbsp brown sugar
- 1/4 tsp cinnamon
- 1/4 tsp vanilla extract
- 2 tbsp water

Procedure

1. Cook the bananas: In a small skillet, melt the butter over medium heat. Add the brown sugar, cinnamon, and water, stirring until the sugar dissolves.

2. Add the bananas: Add the sliced bananas to the skillet and cook for about 3-4 minutes, until the bananas soften and are coated with the sauce.

3. Blend or mash: Transfer the cooked bananas to a blender or food processor and blend until smooth, or mash with a fork for a chunkier texture.

4. Add the vanilla extract, stir, and serve warm.

Pineapple Tapioca Pudding

Prep Time: 10 mins | Cook Time: 25 mins | Serves: 4

Per Serving: Calories: 190 | Fat: 4g | Carbs: 36g | Fiber: 1g | Protein: 3g

Ingredients

- 1/4 cup small tapioca pearls
- 2 cups milk
- 1/2 cup crushed pineapple (canned in juice)
- 1/4 cup sugar
- 1/2 tsp vanilla extract

Procedure

1. Cook the tapioca: In a saucepan, combine the milk and tapioca pearls. Bring to a simmer over medium heat, stirring frequently to prevent sticking. Cook for 20-25 minutes until the tapioca pearls become translucent and soft.

2. Add sugar and vanilla: Stir in the sugar and vanilla extract, and cook for an additional 2 minutes.

3. Combine with pineapple: Remove from heat and fold in the crushed pineapple.

4. Serve warm or chilled. The pudding should be soft and easy to swallow.

Berries with Vanilla Custard

Prep Time: 10 mins | Cook Time: 10 mins | Serves: 4

Per Serving: Calories: 160 | Fat: 5g | Carbs: 28g | Fiber: 3g | Protein: 3g

Ingredients

- 1 cup mixed berries (such as strawberries, blueberries, or raspberries, minced or soft)
- 1 cup milk
- 2 egg yolks
- 1/4 cup sugar
- 1 tsp vanilla extract

Procedure

1. Prepare the custard: In a small saucepan, heat the milk over medium heat until warm. In a separate bowl, whisk together the egg yolks and sugar. Gradually pour the warm milk into the egg mixture, whisking constantly.

2. Cook the custard: Pour the mixture back into the saucepan and cook over low heat, stirring constantly, until the custard thickens (about 5 minutes). Remove from heat and stir in the vanilla extract.

3. Mince or mash the berries as needed, then serve them topped with the warm or chilled vanilla custard.

Minced Soft Macaroni and Cheese Bites

Prep Time: 10 mins | Cook Time: 20 mins | Serves: 4

Per Serving: Calories: 250 | Fat: 12g | Carbs: 30g | Fiber: 1g | Protein: 8g

Ingredients

- 1 1/2 cups cooked macaroni (very soft)
- 1/2 cup shredded cheese (cheddar or mozzarella)
- 1/4 cup breadcrumbs (softened)
- 1 egg, beaten
- 1 tbsp butter
- Salt and pepper to taste

Procedure

1. Preheat the oven: Preheat your oven to 350°F (175°C).

2. Combine ingredients: In a bowl, combine the cooked macaroni, shredded cheese, softened breadcrumbs, beaten egg, butter, salt, and pepper. Stir until fully mixed.

3. Form bites: Scoop out small portions of the mixture and form them into soft bites.

4. Bake: Place the bites on a greased baking sheet and bake for 15-20 minutes, until golden brown and set.

5. Let cool slightly and serve. Mince or mash the bites further for easier chewing if necessary.

Meal plan

Day 1

- Day 1Breakfast: Mashed Berry Parfait with Soft Oats Layers
- Lunch: Minced Shepherd's Pie
- Dinner: Minced Soft Beef Stroganoff with Soft Noodles
- Snack: Soft Baked Apple Slices

Day 2

- Breakfast: Minced Egg and Cheese Breakfast Burrito
- Lunch: Soft Lentil and Vegetable Soup
- Dinner: Minced Chicken with Olive Tapenade
- Snack: Honeyed Pear Purée

Day 3

- Breakfast: Turkey Sausage with Soft Polenta
- Lunch: Minced Soft Beef Tacos
- Dinner: Minced Turkey Shepherd's Pie
- Snack: Pineapple Tapioca Pudding

Day 4

- Breakfast: Minced Soft Baked Apples with Cinnamon
- Lunch: Minced Vegetable Stir-fry with Soft Tofu
- Dinner: Minced Soft Meat Lasagna
- Snack: Minced Soft Macaroni and Cheese Bites

Day 5

- Breakfast: Minced Huevos Rancheros with Avocado
- Lunch: Soft Barley and Mushroom Soup
- Dinner: Seafood Chowder Soup
- Snack: Banana Foster Purée

Day 6

- Breakfast: Minced Tofu Scramble with Soft Veggies
- Lunch: Minced Chicken Alfredo with Softened Pasta
- Dinner: Minced Soft Turkey with Stuffing and Gravy
- Snack: Berries with Vanilla Custard

Day 7

- Breakfast: Minced Sweet Potato Hash with Soft Poached Eggs
- Lunch: Mashed Bean and Vegetable Casserole
- Dinner: Minced Chicken and Dumplings
- Snack: Minced Soft Fruit Smoothie

Dysphagia cookbook for beginners

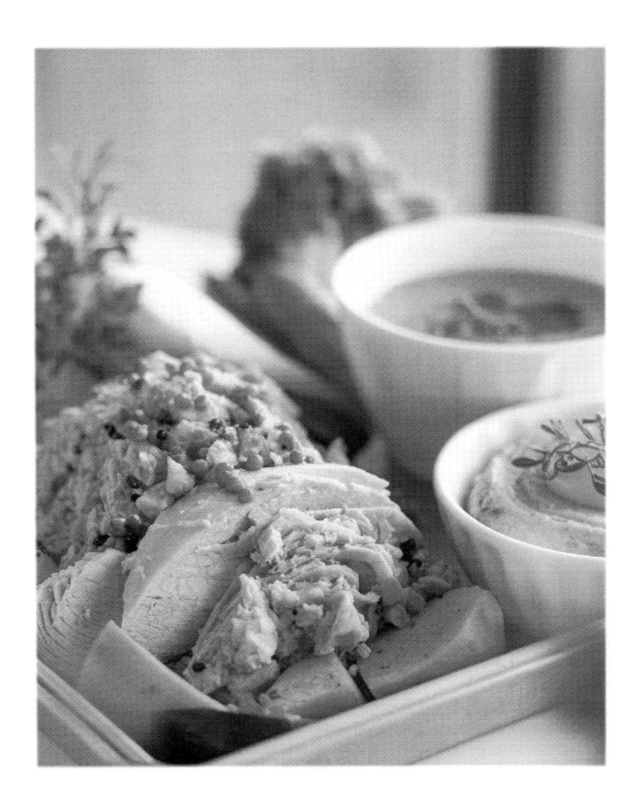

Dysphagia cookbook for beginners

Chapter 5

Level 3: Advanced/Soft-Solid Foods (Soft, Easy-to-Chew, Near-Normal)

Soft Scrambled Eggs with Toast

Prep Time: 5 mins | Cook Time: 5 mins | Serves: 2
Per Serving: Calories: 220 | Fat: 14g | Carbs: 12g | Fiber: 2g | Protein: 12g

Ingredients

- 4 eggs
- 2 tbsp milk
- 1 tbsp butter
- 2 slices of soft bread (lightly toasted)
- Salt and pepper to taste

Procedure

1. Prepare the eggs: In a bowl, whisk the eggs with the milk until well combined.

2. Cook the eggs: Melt butter in a non-stick pan over low heat. Add the eggs and cook slowly, stirring gently, until soft and creamy.

3. Lightly toast the bread: Toast the bread until just barely crispy, making sure it is still soft enough to chew easily.

4. Serve the scrambled eggs alongside the soft toast. Cut the toast into small, easy-to-chew pieces if necessary.

Soft Pancakes with Syrup and Softened Fruit

Prep Time: 10 mins | Cook Time: 15 mins | Serves: 4
Per Serving: Calories: 280 | Fat: 8g | Carbs: 45g | Fiber: 2g | Protein: 6g

Ingredients

- 1 cup all-purpose flour
- 1 tbsp sugar
- 1 tsp baking powder
- 1 egg
- 1 cup milk
- 1 tbsp butter (melted)
- 1/2 cup softened fruit (such as peaches, bananas, or berries)
- Maple syrup for serving

Procedure

1. Prepare the pancake batter: In a bowl, whisk together the flour, sugar, and baking powder. In a separate bowl, whisk the egg, milk, and melted butter. Gradually mix the wet ingredients into the dry ingredients.

2. Cook the pancakes: Heat a non-stick skillet over medium heat. Pour small amounts of the batter onto the skillet and cook for 2-3 minutes on each side until golden brown and cooked through.

3. Soften the fruit: If needed, microwave the fruit for 30 seconds to soften it further.

4. Serve the soft pancakes with syrup and softened fruit on the side.

Dysphagia cookbook for beginners

Cream of Sweet Potato Soup

Prep Time: 10 mins | Cook Time: 20 mins | Serves: 4

Per Serving: Calories: 180 | Fat: 6g | Carbs: 30g | Fiber: 4g | Protein: 3g

Ingredients

- 2 large sweet potatoes, peeled and cubed
- 1 small onion, chopped
- 2 cups low-sodium vegetable broth
- 1/2 cup cream
- 1 tbsp butter
- Salt and pepper to taste

Procedure

1. Cook the vegetables: In a large pot, sauté the onions in butter until soft. Add the sweet potatoes and broth. Bring to a boil, then reduce heat and simmer for 15 minutes, or until the sweet potatoes are soft.

2. Blend the soup: Transfer the mixture to a blender and blend until smooth. Stir in the cream.

3. Season with salt and pepper, and serve warm.

Soft Omelette with Minced Vegetables and Cheese

Prep Time: 10 mins | Cook Time: 5 mins | Serves: 2

Per Serving: Calories: 250 | Fat: 18g | Carbs: 4g | Fiber: 1g | Protein: 16g

Ingredients

- 4 eggs
- 1/4 cup finely minced vegetables (such as bell peppers, spinach, or onions)
- 1/4 cup shredded cheese (cheddar or mozzarella)
- 1 tbsp butter
- Salt and pepper to taste

Procedure

1. Prepare the eggs: Whisk the eggs in a bowl until well combined.

2. Cook the omelette: Heat butter in a non-stick skillet over medium heat. Pour in the eggs, then sprinkle the minced vegetables and cheese evenly over the top. Cook for 2-3 minutes until set, then fold the omelette in half.

3. Serve warm with a side of soft toast or softened fruit, if desired.

Dysphagia cookbook for beginners

Smoked Salmon, Egg, and Avocado Mash Sandwich

Prep Time: 10 mins | Cook Time: 5 mins | Serves: 2

Per Serving: Calories: 320 | Fat: 18g | Carbs: 28g | Fiber: 4g | Protein: 15g

Ingredients

- 2 soft slices of sandwich bread
- 1 ripe avocado, mashed
- 2 hard-boiled eggs, mashed
- 2 slices of smoked salmon (optional)
- 1 tbsp lemon juice
- Salt and pepper to taste

Procedure

1. Prepare the mash: In a bowl, mash the avocado and hard-boiled eggs together. Add the lemon juice, salt, and pepper, and mix well.

2. Assemble the sandwich: Spread the avocado and egg mixture onto one slice of bread, top with smoked salmon, and place the second slice of bread on top.

3. Cut the sandwich into small, manageable pieces if needed.

Egg and Avocado Mash

Prep Time: 5 mins | Cook Time: 10 mins | Serves: 2

Per Serving: Calories: 260 | Fat: 18g | Carbs: 14g | Fiber: 6g | Protein: 10g

Ingredients

- 2 hard-boiled eggs, mashed
- 1 ripe avocado, mashed
- 1 tbsp lemon juice
- Salt and pepper to taste

Procedure

1. Prepare the eggs: Mash the hard-boiled eggs in a bowl.

2. Prepare the avocado: In a separate bowl, mash the avocado and mix in the lemon juice, salt, and pepper.

3. Mix the mashed eggs with the avocado and serve as a topping for toast or eat on its own.

Dysphagia cookbook for beginners

Breakfast Burrito with Scrambled Eggs and Softened Sausage

Prep Time: 10 mins | Cook Time: 10 mins | Serves: 2
Per Serving: Calories: 350 | Fat: 20g | Carbs: 25g | Fiber: 2g | Protein: 18g

Ingredients

- 4 eggs
- 2 soft flour tortillas
- 1/4 cup shredded cheese
- 2 small sausage links, softened (boiled or cooked gently until soft)
- 1 tbsp butter
- Salt and pepper to taste

Procedure

1. Prepare the scrambled eggs: Whisk the eggs in a bowl. Melt butter in a skillet over medium heat and cook the eggs until soft and scrambled.

2. Soften the sausage: Boil or gently cook the sausages until soft, then slice into small, easy-to-chew pieces.

3. Assemble the burrito: On each tortilla, place half the scrambled eggs, cheese, and softened sausage pieces.

4. Fold the tortilla into a burrito shape, cutting into small pieces if needed for easier chewing. Serve warm.

Soft Poached Eggs with Soft Hash Browns

Prep Time: 10 mins | Cook Time: 20 mins | Serves: 2

Per Serving: Calories: 300 | Fat: 15g | Carbs: 30g | Fiber: 3g | Protein: 10g

Ingredients

- 4 eggs

- 2 medium potatoes, peeled and grated

- 2 tbsp olive oil

- Salt and pepper to taste

Procedure

1. Prepare the hash browns: Grate the potatoes and press out any excess moisture. Heat olive oil in a skillet over medium heat, add the grated potatoes, and cook for 8-10 minutes, flipping halfway, until golden brown and soft.

2. Poach the eggs: In a small pot, bring water to a simmer. Crack the eggs into the water and poach for 3-4 minutes, until the whites are set but the yolks remain soft.

3. Serve the soft poached eggs on top of the soft hash browns. Season with salt and pepper to taste.

Lemon Chickpea and Tahini Dip with Soft Bread

Prep Time: 10 mins | Cook Time: 0 mins | Serves: 4

Per Serving: Calories: 250 | Fat: 12g | Carbs: 30g | Fiber: 8g | Protein: 8g

Ingredients

- 1 can (15 oz) chickpeas, rinsed and drained
- 2 tbsp tahini
- 1 tbsp olive oil
- 1 tbsp lemon juice
- 1/2 tsp garlic powder
- Salt and pepper to taste
- Soft bread for serving (lightly toasted if desired)

Procedure

1. Prepare the dip: In a blender or food processor, combine the chickpeas, tahini, olive oil, lemon juice, garlic powder, salt, and pepper. Blend until smooth and creamy.

2. Serve the dip with soft bread or lightly toasted bread, cut into small, manageable pieces. You can also serve with softened vegetables like cucumbers or steamed carrots.

Creamy Coconut and Pineapple Rice

Prep Time: 5 mins | Cook Time: 20 mins | Serves: 4

Per Serving: Calories: 280 | Fat: 12g | Carbs: 40g | Fiber: 3g | Protein: 4g

Ingredients

- 1 cup white rice
- 1/2 cup coconut milk
- 1/2 cup crushed pineapple (canned in juice, drained)
- 1 tbsp sugar (optional)
- 1/4 tsp vanilla extract

Procedure

1. Cook the rice: In a pot, cook the rice according to package instructions until tender.

2. Add the coconut milk: Once the rice is cooked, stir in the coconut milk, crushed pineapple, sugar (if using), and vanilla extract. Cook for an additional 2-3 minutes until everything is warmed through.

3. Serve warm as a soft, creamy breakfast or snack. You can garnish with a sprinkle of cinnamon if desired.

Flavorful Lunch

Soft Meatloaf with Mashed Potatoes

Prep Time: 20 mins | Cook Time: 40 mins | Serves: 4

Per Serving: Calories: 350 | Fat: 18g | Carbs: 35g | Fiber: 4g | Protein: 20g

Ingredients

- 1 lb ground beef or turkey
- 1/2 cup breadcrumbs (softened)
- 1 egg, beaten
- 1/4 cup milk
- 1 tbsp ketchup
- 2 large potatoes, peeled and chopped
- 1 tbsp butter
- 1/4 cup milk (for mashed potatoes)
- Salt and pepper to taste

Procedure

1. Prepare the meatloaf mixture: In a mixing bowl, combine the ground meat, softened breadcrumbs, beaten egg, milk, ketchup, salt, and pepper. Mix well.

2. Form the meatloaf: Shape the mixture into a loaf and place in a greased loaf pan.

3. Bake the meatloaf: Bake at 350°F (175°C) for 35-40 minutes until fully cooked.

4. Prepare the mashed potatoes: While the meatloaf is baking, boil the chopped potatoes until tender, about 15 minutes. Drain and mash with butter and milk.

5. Serve the soft meatloaf alongside the mashed potatoes.

Shredded Chicken Wrap with Soft Tortilla

Prep Time: 10 mins | Cook Time: 15 mins | Serves: 2

Per Serving: Calories: 300 | Fat: 12g | Carbs: 25g | Fiber: 3g | Protein: 20g

Ingredients

- 1 cooked chicken breast, shredded
- 2 soft flour tortillas
- 1/4 cup shredded cheese
- 1 tbsp mayonnaise
- 1 tbsp sour cream (optional)
- Salt and pepper to taste

Procedure

1. Shred the chicken: Use two forks to shred the cooked chicken breast into small, soft pieces.
2. Assemble the wrap: On each tortilla, spread mayonnaise and sour cream, then add the shredded chicken and cheese.
3. Fold the tortilla into a wrap. Cut into small pieces for easier chewing if needed.

Creamy Poached Crab Salad

Prep Time: 10 mins | Cook Time: 10 mins | Serves: 2

Per Serving: Calories: 250 | Fat: 15g | Carbs: 10g | Fiber: 2g | Protein: 20g

Ingredients

- 1/2 lb crab meat (fresh or canned, drained)
- 1/4 cup mayonnaise
- 1 tbsp lemon juice
- 1/2 tsp Dijon mustard
- 1 tbsp chopped soft herbs (such as parsley or dill)
- Salt and pepper to taste

Procedure

1. Prepare the salad: In a bowl, gently mix the crab meat, mayonnaise, lemon juice, mustard, and herbs until well combined.
2. Poach the crab meat (if fresh): If using fresh crab, poach in simmering water for 3-4 minutes until cooked, then drain.
3. Serve the crab salad chilled or at room temperature with soft bread or crackers.

Dysphagia cookbook for beginners

Soft Chicken Salad Sandwich on Soft Bread

Prep Time: 10 mins | Cook Time: 0 mins | Serves: 2

Per Serving: Calories: 300 | Fat: 15g | Carbs: 30g | Fiber: 2g | Protein: 15g

Ingredients

- 1 cooked chicken breast, shredded
- 2 tbsp mayonnaise
- 1 tbsp plain yogurt
- 1 tsp Dijon mustard
- 4 slices of soft sandwich bread
- 1 tbsp finely chopped celery (optional)
- Salt and pepper to taste

Procedure

1. Prepare the chicken salad: In a bowl, mix the shredded chicken, mayonnaise, yogurt, mustard, and celery (if using). Season with salt and pepper.

2. Assemble the sandwich: Spread the chicken salad on two slices of soft bread and top with the remaining slices.

3. Cut the sandwich into small, manageable pieces if needed.

Soft Baked Fish with Soft Vegetables

Prep Time: 10 mins | Cook Time: 20 mins | Serves: 2

Per Serving: Calories: 250 | Fat: 10g | Carbs: 20g | Fiber: 4g | Protein: 25g

Ingredients

- 2 fillets of soft white fish (such as cod or haddock)
- 1 tbsp olive oil
- 1 lemon, sliced
- 1 cup soft vegetables (such as carrots or zucchini), steamed
- Salt and pepper to taste

Procedure

1. Prepare the fish: Preheat the oven to 375°F (190°C). Place the fish fillets on a baking sheet lined with parchment paper. Drizzle with olive oil and top with lemon slices.

2. Bake the fish: Bake for 15-20 minutes, or until the fish is soft and flakes easily with a fork.

3. Steam the vegetables: While the fish is baking, steam the soft vegetables until tender.

4. Serve the baked fish with the steamed vegetables on the side.

Soft Baked Potato with Softened Sour Cream and Cheese

Prep Time: 5 mins | Cook Time: 45 mins | Serves: 2

Per Serving: Calories: 250 | Fat: 10g | Carbs: 35g | Fiber: 5g | Protein: 6g

Ingredients

- 2 medium russet potatoes
- 1/4 cup sour cream (softened)
- 1/4 cup shredded cheddar cheese
- 1 tbsp butter
- Salt and pepper to taste

Procedure

1. Bake the potatoes: Preheat the oven to 400°F (200°C). Poke a few holes in each potato with a fork and bake directly on the oven rack for 45 minutes, or until soft.

2. Soften the sour cream: If needed, microwave the sour cream for 10 seconds to ensure it's soft and easy to mix.

3. Assemble: Split each baked potato open and fluff the inside with a fork. Add butter, softened sour cream, and shredded cheese.

4. Serve warm, and mash further if needed for easier chewing.

Soft Chicken Quesadilla with Softened Refried Beans

Prep Time: 10 mins | Cook Time: 10 mins | Serves: 2

Per Serving: Calories: 350 | Fat: 16g | Carbs: 32g | Fiber: 6g | Protein: 18g

Ingredients

- 1 cooked chicken breast, shredded
- 2 soft flour tortillas
- 1/2 cup refried beans (softened)
- 1/4 cup shredded cheese
- 1 tbsp olive oil

Procedure

1. Prepare the quesadilla: Spread softened refried beans on one tortilla. Add shredded chicken and cheese. Place the second tortilla on top.
2. Cook the quesadilla: Heat olive oil in a skillet over medium heat. Cook the quesadilla for 3-4 minutes on each side until the cheese melts and the tortilla is lightly golden.
3. Serve: Cut into small, easy-to-chew pieces and serve warm.

Soft Turkey and Soft Mashed Sweet Potatoes

Prep Time: 10 mins | Cook Time: 30 mins | Serves: 2

Per Serving: Calories: 280 | Fat: 8g | Carbs: 35g | Fiber: 5g | Protein: 20g

Ingredients

- 1/2 lb cooked turkey breast, sliced thin or minced
- 2 medium sweet potatoes, peeled and chopped
- 1 tbsp butter
- 1/4 cup milk
- Salt and pepper to taste

Procedure

1. Cook the sweet potatoes: Boil the sweet potatoes in a pot of water for 15-20 minutes until soft. Drain and mash with butter and milk until smooth.
2. Prepare the turkey: Slice or mince the cooked turkey breast into small, soft pieces.
3. Serve: Serve the soft turkey with the mashed sweet potatoes. Season with salt and pepper to taste.

117

Chickpea Spinach Curry

Prep Time: 10 mins | Cook Time: 20 mins | Serves: 4

Per Serving: Calories: 300 | Fat: 10g | Carbs: 40g | Fiber: 10g | Protein: 10g

Ingredients

- 1 can chickpeas, rinsed and mashed slightly
- 2 cups fresh spinach (cooked and finely minced)
- 1 small onion, finely chopped
- 1 tbsp curry powder
- 1/2 cup coconut milk
- 1 tbsp olive oil
- Salt and pepper to taste

Procedure

1. Cook the onion: In a large skillet, heat olive oil over medium heat. Add the onion and sauté for 5 minutes until soft.

2. Add the chickpeas and spinach: Stir in the chickpeas, spinach, and curry powder. Cook for another 5 minutes.

3. Add coconut milk: Pour in the coconut milk and simmer for 5-7 minutes until the mixture thickens.

4. Serve warm, optionally with soft rice or naan.

Dysphagia cookbook for beginners

Garlic Butter White Bean Mash with Soft Carrot

Prep Time: 10 mins | Cook Time: 15 mins | Serves: 2

Per Serving: Calories: 240 | Fat: 8g | Carbs: 35g | Fiber: 8g | Protein: 10g

Ingredients

- 1 can white beans (such as cannellini), drained and rinsed
- 2 medium carrots, peeled and chopped
- 1 tbsp butter
- 1 clove garlic, minced
- 1/4 cup vegetable broth
- Salt and pepper to taste

Procedure

1. Cook the carrots: Boil the chopped carrots in water for 10-12 minutes until soft. Drain and set aside.

2. Prepare the white bean mash: In a saucepan, melt butter over medium heat and sauté the garlic for 1-2 minutes. Add the beans and vegetable broth, and cook for 5 minutes. Mash the beans with a fork or potato masher until smooth.

3. Serve the white bean mash with the soft-cooked carrots on the side.

Dinner ideas

Soft Beef Stroganoff with Soft Noodles

Prep Time: 15 mins | Cook Time: 30 mins | Serves: 4

Per Serving: Calories: 400 | Fat: 20g | Carbs: 35g | Fiber: 4g | Protein: 25g

Ingredients

- 1 lb ground beef, minced or very finely chopped
- 1 small onion, minced
- 1/2 cup mushrooms, minced
- 1 cup sour cream
- 1/4 cup beef broth
- 6 oz soft egg noodles, cooked until very soft
- 1 tbsp olive oil
- Salt and pepper to taste

Procedure

1. Cook the beef: In a large skillet, heat the olive oil over medium heat. Add the minced beef, onion, and mushrooms, cooking until the meat is browned and the vegetables are softened (about 10 minutes).

2. Make the sauce: Stir in the beef broth and sour cream. Simmer for 5-7 minutes until the sauce thickens slightly.

3. Cook the noodles: Cook the egg noodles in boiling water until very soft. Drain and set aside.

4. Add the soft noodles to the beef mixture and toss to coat. Serve warm.

Soft Pasta with Pureed Meat Sauce

Prep Time: 10 mins | Cook Time: 20 mins | Serves: 4

Per Serving: Calories: 350 | Fat: 12g | Carbs: 40g | Fiber: 4g | Protein: 20g

Ingredients

- 8 oz soft pasta (such as penne or fusilli)

- 1 lb ground beef or turkey

- 1 cup marinara sauce (smooth)

- 1/2 cup vegetable broth

- 1 tbsp olive oil

- 1/4 cup grated Parmesan cheese

- Salt and pepper to taste

Procedure

1. Cook the pasta: Boil the pasta until very soft (beyond al dente). Drain and set aside.

2. Prepare the meat sauce: In a skillet, cook the ground beef or turkey in olive oil over medium heat until fully cooked. Add the marinara sauce and broth, then blend or puree the meat mixture until smooth.

3. Toss the softened pasta with the pureed meat sauce. Sprinkle with grated Parmesan and serve.

Soft Pork Chops with Softened Rice and Gravy

Prep Time: 10 mins | Cook Time: 30 mins | Serves: 4

Per Serving: Calories: 400 | Fat: 18g | Carbs: 35g | Fiber: 3g | Protein: 30g

Ingredients

- 4 boneless pork chops, cooked until very soft
- 1 cup cooked white rice (very soft)
- 1 cup gravy (smooth, no lumps)
- 1 tbsp olive oil
- Salt and pepper to taste

Procedure

1. Cook the pork chops: Season the pork chops with salt and pepper. Heat olive oil in a skillet and cook the pork chops over low heat for 20-25 minutes, until they are tender and easy to chew.

2. Cook the rice: Boil the rice until very soft, then drain and set aside.

3. Serve the pork chops with softened rice and smooth gravy on top.

Soft Baked Lasagna with Soft Ricotta Filling

Prep Time: 20 mins | Cook Time: 40 mins | Serves: 4

Per Serving: Calories: 450 | Fat: 20g | Carbs: 40g | Fiber: 5g | Protein: 25g

Ingredients

- 6 soft lasagna noodles, cooked until very soft
- 1 lb ground beef or turkey, minced
- 1 cup marinara sauce (smooth)
- 1/2 cup ricotta cheese
- 1/4 cup shredded mozzarella cheese
- 1 tbsp olive oil
- Salt and pepper to taste

Procedure

1. Cook the lasagna noodles: Boil the lasagna noodles until very soft. Drain and set aside.

2. Prepare the meat sauce: In a skillet, cook the minced ground meat with olive oil until browned. Stir in the marinara sauce and simmer for 5 minutes.

3. Assemble the lasagna: In a greased baking dish, layer the soft lasagna noodles, ricotta cheese, and meat sauce. Repeat the layers and top with mozzarella.

4. Bake: Preheat the oven to 350°F (175°C) and bake for 25-30 minutes, until the cheese is melted and bubbly.

5. Let cool slightly before serving. Cut into small pieces for easier chewing.

Soft Chicken Pot Pie with Soft Crust and Minced Veggies

Prep Time: 20 mins | Cook Time: 35 mins | Serves: 4

Per Serving: Calories: 400 | Fat: 20g | Carbs: 40g | Fiber: 5g | Protein: 25g

Ingredients

- 1 lb cooked chicken breast, minced

- 1 cup mixed soft vegetables (carrots, peas, potatoes), minced

- 1/2 cup low-sodium chicken broth

- 1/4 cup heavy cream

- 1 pre-made soft pie crust

- 1 tbsp butter

Procedure

1. Prepare the filling: In a skillet, melt the butter over medium heat. Add the minced chicken and vegetables, then stir in the chicken broth and heavy cream. Simmer for 5 minutes.

2. Assemble the pie: Pour the chicken mixture into a greased pie dish. Place the soft pie crust on top and crimp the edges.

3. Bake: Preheat the oven to 350°F (175°C) and bake for 25-30 minutes, until the crust is golden and the filling is heated through.

4. Let cool slightly before serving.

Soft Turkey with Softened Stuffing and Gravy

Prep Time: 15 mins | Cook Time: 30 mins | Serves: 4

Per Serving: Calories: 380 | Fat: 14g | Carbs: 40g | Fiber: 4g | Protein: 25g

Ingredients

- 1 lb cooked turkey breast, sliced thin
- 1 cup softened stuffing (prepared with extra broth for moisture)
- 1 cup gravy (smooth, no lumps)
- 1 tbsp olive oil
- Salt and pepper to taste

Procedure

1. Prepare the stuffing: Prepare the stuffing according to package directions, adding extra broth to ensure it is very soft and moist.

2. Cook the turkey: Slice the cooked turkey breast into thin, soft slices.

3. Serve: Serve the turkey with softened stuffing and gravy on top.

Soft Shepherd's Pie with Soft Mashed Potatoes and Minced Meat

Prep Time: 20 mins | Cook Time: 40 mins | Serves: 4

Per Serving: Calories: 350 | Fat: 15g | Carbs: 40g | Fiber: 5g | Protein: 20g

Ingredients

- 1 lb ground beef or turkey, minced

- 1 cup soft mixed vegetables (peas, carrots, corn), minced

- 2 medium potatoes, peeled and chopped

- 1 tbsp butter

- 1/4 cup milk

- Salt and pepper to taste

Procedure

1. Prepare the mashed potatoes: Boil the potatoes in a large pot of water until tender, about 15 minutes. Drain and mash with butter and milk until smooth.

2. Cook the meat: In a skillet, cook the minced meat over medium heat until browned. Add the minced vegetables and simmer for 5 minutes. Season with salt and pepper.

3. Assemble the pie: In a baking dish, spread the minced meat and vegetable mixture. Top with the mashed potatoes.

4. Bake: Preheat the oven to 350°F (175°C) and bake for 20-25 minutes, until the top is golden.

5. Serve warm, ensuring the dish is soft and easy to chew.

Soft Vegetable Stir-fry with Soft Tofu and Softened Rice

Prep Time: 10 mins | Cook Time: 15 mins | Serves: 4

Per Serving: Calories: 280 | Fat: 12g | Carbs: 35g | Fiber: 6g | Protein: 10g

Ingredients

- 1 block soft tofu, cubed

- 1 cup soft vegetables (such as zucchini, carrots, and bell peppers), minced

- 1 tbsp soy sauce

- 1 tbsp olive oil

- 2 cups cooked soft rice

- 1/4 tsp ginger (optional)

Procedure

1. Cook the tofu: In a skillet, heat olive oil over medium heat. Add the tofu and cook for 3-4 minutes until lightly golden.

2. Sauté the vegetables: Add the minced vegetables and ginger (if using) to the skillet. Stir-fry for 5-7 minutes until the vegetables are tender.

3. Add soy sauce: Stir in the soy sauce and cook for another 1-2 minutes.

4. Serve the stir-fried vegetables and tofu over softened rice.

Soft Baked Ziti with Soft Meat Sauce and Melted Cheese

Prep Time: 20 mins | Cook Time: 30 mins | Serves: 4

Per Serving: Calories: 450 | Fat: 20g | Carbs: 50g | Fiber: 6g | Protein: 25g

Ingredients

- 8 oz ziti pasta, cooked until very soft
- 1 lb ground beef or turkey, minced
- 1 cup marinara sauce (smooth)
- 1/2 cup ricotta cheese
- 1/2 cup shredded mozzarella cheese
- 1 tbsp olive oil
- Salt and pepper to taste

Procedure

1. Cook the pasta: Boil the ziti pasta until very soft, then drain and set aside.

2. Prepare the meat sauce: In a skillet, cook the minced ground meat in olive oil until browned. Stir in the marinara sauce and simmer for 5 minutes.

3. Assemble the ziti: In a greased baking dish, mix the soft ziti pasta with the meat sauce. Add dollops of ricotta cheese on top and sprinkle with mozzarella.

4. Bake: Preheat the oven to 350°F (175°C) and bake for 20-25 minutes, until the cheese is melted and bubbly.

5. Let cool slightly before serving, ensuring the dish is soft enough for easy chewing.

Soft Chicken Fajitas with Soft Tortillas and Softened Peppers

Prep Time: 15 mins | Cook Time: 15 mins | Serves: 4

Per Serving: Calories: 350 | Fat: 12g | Carbs: 35g | Fiber: 5g | Protein: 20g

Ingredients

- 2 chicken breasts, cooked and shredded
- 1/2 cup softened bell peppers (minced)
- 1/2 onion, minced
- 1 tbsp olive oil
- 4 soft flour tortillas
- 1/4 cup shredded cheese
- Salt and pepper to taste

Procedure

1. Cook the vegetables: In a skillet, heat the olive oil over medium heat. Add the minced peppers and onions, cooking for 5-7 minutes until softened.

2. Shred the chicken: Add the shredded chicken to the skillet and cook for another 2-3 minutes, stirring to combine. Season with salt and pepper.

3. Assemble the fajitas: Warm the tortillas and fill them with the chicken and softened vegetables. Sprinkle with shredded cheese.

4. Fold the tortillas and cut into small pieces if needed for easier chewing.

Snacks and Light Meals

Ripe Fruit Smoothies

Prep Time: 5 mins | Cook Time: 0 mins | Serves: 2

Per Serving: Calories: 180 | Fat: 3g | Carbs: 35g | Fiber: 4g | Protein: 5g

Ingredients

- 1 ripe banana
- 1/2 cup ripe strawberries (or any soft fruit)
- 1/2 cup yogurt (or milk)
- 1 tbsp honey (optional)
- 1/4 tsp vanilla extract (optional)

Procedure

1. Blend the fruits: Place the banana, strawberries, yogurt (or milk), and honey into a blender. Blend until smooth.
2. Pour the smoothie into glasses and serve immediately. Adjust the thickness with more milk or yogurt if necessary.

Soft Cheese and Crackers

Prep Time: 5 mins | Cook Time: 0 mins | Serves: 2

Per Serving: Calories: 150 | Fat: 10g | Carbs: 12g | Fiber: 1g | Protein: 6g

Ingredients

- 1/4 cup soft cheese (such as cream cheese or brie)
- 6 soft crackers (or softened whole wheat crackers)
- Optional: Sliced soft fruit (such as pear or apple slices)

Procedure

1. Serve the cheese: Spread the soft cheese on the crackers.
2. Optional topping: Top with a thin slice of soft fruit, such as pear or apple.
3. Serve immediately. Ensure the crackers are softened if needed for easier chewing.

Soft Cake with Blended Fruit

Prep Time: 10 mins | Cook Time: 30 mins | Serves: 6

Per Serving: Calories: 250 | Fat: 12g | Carbs: 30g | Fiber: 2g | Protein: 4g

Ingredients

- 1 soft sponge cake (pre-made or homemade)
- 1 cup ripe fruit (such as peaches, strawberries, or raspberries)
- 1/4 cup sugar (optional)
- 1/4 cup water

Procedure

1. Prepare the fruit: Blend the ripe fruit with water and sugar (if using) until smooth.

2. Prepare the cake: Cut the soft sponge cake into small pieces.

3. Serve the sponge cake with the blended fruit purée drizzled on top for extra moisture and flavor.

Fruit Tart Purée

Prep Time: 10 mins | Cook Time: 10 mins | Serves: 4

Per Serving: Calories: 200 | Fat: 8g | Carbs: 30g | Fiber: 2g | Protein: 3g

Ingredients

- 1 cup mixed berries (such as strawberries, raspberries, and blueberries)
- 1/4 cup water
- 1 tbsp honey
- 1/4 tsp vanilla extract
- 4 small tart shells (store-bought or homemade, softened if needed)

Procedure

1. Prepare the purée: In a small saucepan, combine the berries, water, honey, and vanilla. Cook over medium heat for 5-7 minutes, stirring frequently, until the berries soften. Remove from heat and blend the mixture until smooth.

2. Assemble the tart: Spoon the fruit purée into the tart shells.

3. Serve the tart warm or chilled.

Dysphagia cookbook for beginners

Soft Sponge Macaron Cake

Prep Time: 15 mins | Cook Time: 25 mins | Serves: 4

Per Serving: Calories: 270 | Fat: 14g | Carbs: 30g | Fiber: 2g | Protein: 5g

Ingredients

- 1/2 cup almond flour
- 1/2 cup powdered sugar
- 2 large eggs (separated)
- 1/4 cup sugar
- 1 tsp vanilla extract
- 1/4 cup whipped cream (optional for serving)

Procedure

1. Prepare the batter: In a mixing bowl, combine almond flour and powdered sugar. In another bowl, whisk the egg whites until soft peaks form. Gradually add sugar while whisking. Fold in the egg yolks, vanilla extract, and almond flour mixture until smooth.

2. Bake: Preheat the oven to 350°F (175°C). Pour the batter into a greased cake pan and bake for 20-25 minutes until the cake is lightly golden.

3. Once the cake has cooled slightly, serve soft slices with whipped cream on top if desired.

Soft Cheese and Soft Crackers

Prep Time: 5 mins | Cook Time: 0 mins | Serves: 2

Per Serving: Calories: 150 | Fat: 10g | Carbs: 12g | Fiber: 1g | Protein: 6g

Ingredients

- 1/4 cup soft cheese (such as cream cheese, goat cheese, or brie)
- 6 soft crackers (or softened whole wheat crackers)
- Optional: Soft fruit slices (such as pears or apples)

Procedure

1. Spread the cheese: Spread the soft cheese on the crackers.
2. Add fruit (optional): Add a thin slice of soft fruit on top for extra flavor and moisture.
3. Serve immediately, ensuring the crackers are softened if needed for easier chewing.

Soft Yogurt with Soft Granola

Prep Time: 5 mins | Cook Time: 0 mins | Serves: 2

Per Serving: Calories: 180 | Fat: 6g | Carbs: 24g | Fiber: 3g | Protein: 8g

Ingredients

- 1 cup plain or vanilla yogurt
- 1/4 cup soft granola (look for soft, chewy granola rather than crunchy varieties)
- 1 tbsp honey (optional)
- Soft fruit (such as mashed banana or berries)

Procedure

1. Prepare the yogurt: In a bowl, spoon the yogurt and add the soft granola on top.
2. Add fruit: Top with soft fruits, such as mashed banana or berries, for extra flavor and texture.
3. Drizzle with honey if desired and serve immediately.

Soft Muffins (Blueberry or Banana)

Prep Time: 15 mins | Cook Time: 25 mins | Serves: 6

Per Serving: Calories: 220 | Fat: 10g | Carbs: 30g | Fiber: 2g | Protein: 4g

Ingredients

- 1 1/2 cups all-purpose flour
- 1/2 cup sugar
- 1 tsp baking powder
- 1/2 cup milk
- 1/4 cup melted butter
- 1 egg, beaten
- 1/2 cup fresh blueberries or mashed banana

Procedure

1. Prepare the batter: In a mixing bowl, combine the flour, sugar, and baking powder. In another bowl, mix the milk, melted butter, and beaten egg. Gradually add the wet ingredients to the dry, then gently fold in the blueberries or mashed banana.

2. Bake: Preheat the oven to 350°F (175°C). Spoon the batter into a muffin tin lined with paper cups and bake for 20-25 minutes until a toothpick inserted in the center comes out clean.

3. Serve: Allow the muffins to cool slightly before serving. Ensure they are soft and easy to chew.

Mea plan

Day 1

- Breakfast: Soft Scrambled Eggs with Toast
- Lunch: Shredded Chicken Wrap with Soft Tortilla
- Dinner: Soft Beef Stroganoff with Soft Noodles
- Snack: Soft Cheese and Crackers

Day 2

- Breakfast: Soft Pancakes with Syrup and Softened Fruit
- Lunch: Soft Chicken Salad Sandwich on Soft Bread
- Dinner: Soft Pasta with Pureed Meat Sauce
- Snack: Soft Yogurt with Soft Granola

Day 3

- Breakfast: Smoked Salmon, Egg, and Avocado Mash Sandwich
- Lunch: Soft Baked Fish with Soft Vegetables
- Dinner: Soft Pork Chops with Softened Rice and Gravy
- Snack: Soft Cake with Blended Fruit

Day 4

- Breakfast: Breakfast Burrito with Scrambled Eggs and Softened Sausage
- Lunch: Soft Baked Potato with Softened Sour Cream and Cheese
- Dinner: Soft Baked Lasagna with Soft Ricotta Filling
- Snack: Soft Sponge Macaron Cake

Day 5

- Breakfast: Soft Poached Eggs with Soft Hash Browns
- Lunch: Soft Chicken Quesadilla with Softened Refried Beans
- Dinner: Soft Chicken Pot Pie with Soft Crust and Minced Veggies
- Snack: Soft Muffins (Blueberry or Banana)

Day 6

- Breakfast: Soft Omelette with Minced Vegetables and Cheese
- Lunch: Chickpea Spinach Curry
- Dinner: Soft Shepherd's Pie with Soft Mashed Potatoes and Minced Meat
- Snack: Ripe Fruit Smoothies

Day 7

- Breakfast: Lemon Chickpea and Tahini Dip with Soft Bread
- Lunch: Soft Turkey and Soft Mashed Sweet Potatoes
- Dinner: Soft Baked Ziti with Soft Meat Sauce and Melted Cheese

135

Conclusion

Living with dysphagia can present unique challenges, but with the right knowledge, tools, and recipes, enjoying mealtimes doesn't have to be difficult or restrictive. This cookbook was designed to provide you with a variety of nourishing, flavorful, and safe-to-eat meals that are both practical and delicious. Whether you're just beginning your journey with a modified diet or have been managing dysphagia for years, these recipes offer flexibility and creativity while ensuring that all textures are safe for swallowing.

We've explored everything from thickened smoothies and soft snacks to full meals that cater to different dysphagia levels. With a wide range of breakfast, lunch, dinner, and snack options, you now have a valuable resource to make daily meals both enjoyable and manageable. Importantly, staying hydrated with thickened drinks and teas has been emphasized throughout, as hydration is crucial for maintaining overall health and well-being.

By following the guidelines, making necessary adjustments to textures, and using the essential Ingredients and tools outlined in this book, you're empowered to create meals that not only Meet your dietary needs but also bring comfort and joy to your daily routine. With care, patience, and a little creativity, managing dysphagia can become a more rewarding experience, giving you or your loved ones the ability to enjoy every bite safely and confidently.

Thank you for taking the time to read this book. I hope it has provided you with the guidance and inspiration needed to create safe, delicious meals for yourself or your loved ones. Your journey with dysphagia can be made easier with the right tools and recipes, and I'm grateful to have been a part of that. Wishing you health and happiness at every meal!

Made in United States
Orlando, FL
08 December 2024

55175026R00076